Aesthetic Otoplasty

Thomas Procedures in Facial Plastic Surgery

Aesthetic Otoplasty

Thomas Procedures in Facial Plastic Surgery

Peter A. Adamson MD FRCSC FACS
Professor and Head
Division of Facial Plastic and Reconstructive Surgery
Department of Otolaryngology—Head and Neck Surgery
University of Toronto
Toronto, Ontario, Canada

Jason A. Litner MD FRCSC
Facial Plastic Surgeon
Profiles Beverly Hills
Los Angeles, California, USA

CBS Publishers & Distributors Pvt Ltd

New Delhi • Bengaluru • Pune • Kochi • Chennai
Mumbai • Kolkata • Hyderabad • Patna • Manipal

People's Medical Publishing House—USA, Shelton, Connecticut

People's Medical Publishing House-USA
2 Enterprise Drive, Suite 509
Shelton, CT 06484
Tel: 203-402-0646
Fax: 203-402-0854
E-mail: info@pmph-usa.com

PMPH-USA

11 12 13 14/PMPH/9 8 7 6 5 4 3 2 1
ISBN-13: 978-1-60795-129-2
ISBN-10: 1-60795-129-0

This Edition has been published by special arrangement with PMPH-USA, Ltd
CBS ISBN: 978-81-239-2249-2

Special Indian Edition: 2013

Published by Satish Kumar Jain for

CBS Publishers & Distributors Pvt Ltd
4819/XI Prahlad Street, 24 Ansari Road, Daryaganj, New Delhi 110 002, India.
Ph: 23289259, 23266861, 23266867   Fax: 011-23243014   Website: www.cbspd.com
                                                      e-mail: delhi@cbspd.com; cbspubs@airtelmail.in

Corporate Office: 204 FIE, Industrial Area, Patparganj, Delhi 110 092
Ph: 4934 4934   Fax: 4934 4935   e-mail: publishing@cbspd.com; publicity@cbspd.com

CBS

Branches

- **Bengaluru:** Seema House 2975, 17th Cross, K.R. Road,
  Banasankari 2nd Stage, Bengaluru 560 070, Karnataka
  Ph: +91-80-26771678/79   Fax: +91-80-26771680   e-mail: bangalore@cbspd.com
- **Pune:** Bhuruk Prestige, Sr. No. 52/12/2+1+3/2 Narhe, Haveli
  (Near Katraj-Dehu Road Bypass), Pune 411 041, Maharashtra
  Ph: +91-20-64704058, 64704059, 32342277   Fax: +91-20-24300160   e-mail: pune@cbspd.com
- **Kochi:** 36/14 Kalluvilakam, Lissie Hospital Road, Kochi 682 018, Kerala
  Ph: +91-484-4059061-65   Fax: +91-484-4059065   e-mail: cochin@cbspd.com
- **Chennai:** 20, West Park Road, Shenoy Nagar, Chennai 600 030, Tamil Nadu
  Ph: +91-44-26260666, 26208620   Fax: +91-44-45530020   e-mail: chennai@cbspd.com

Representatives

- **Mumbai** 0-9833017933   • **Kolkata** 0-9831437309   • **Hyderabad** 0-9885175004
- **Patna**   0-9334159340   • **Manipal** 0-9742022075

Printed at R P Printers, Noida

Preface

Otoplasty is often casually approached as a quick and relatively painless procedure, but the surgeon who is most knowledgeable understands the complexity of this 'simple' operation. Overcoming the intrinsic cartilaginous spring of the native auricle to reproduce a naturally symmetrical and stable contour, remains a very challenging proposition. Every good operation begins with a meticulous assessment and assiduous operative planning. Assurance of a satisfactory otoplasty result rests also on fastidious execution of that plan with a view towards reinforcing the stability of the cartilaginous auricular framework. Our graduated technique, starting with conservative postauricular skin excision and conchal setback, and followed by antihelical shaping via precise suture placement, has yielded exceedingly reproducible outcomes and a high degree of patient satifaction in our hands. Supplementary adjustments can then be individualized based on the persistent deformity noted. We reserve cartilage-cutting techniques for the rare instance of a densely thickened or inflexible cartilage that is refractory to cartilage-sparing manipulations.

A formula for enduring success with this fascinating aesthetic procedure combines an appreciation for anatomic nuance with painstaking attention to detail and untiring intraoperative reevaluation. The vast number of known otoplasty methods is a tribute to the level of difficulty involved in this procedure. The objective of this volume is to provide a critical and comprehensive review of the state-of-the-art of our specialty as it relates to cosmetic auricular surgery. It is our hope that this information has been distilled to the extent that surgeons of every experience level may find some surgical pearls within these pages that are of some use to their current and future practice of otoplasty. Whatever the preferred maneuvers, adherence to the goals and principles outlined in this volume will help to circumvent the manifold pitfalls associated with this challenging but rewarding operation.

Peter A. Adamson, MD, FRCSC, FACS
Jason A. Litner, MD, FRCSC

TABLE OF CONTENTS

Introduction

There is no question that, where estimation of facial beauty is concerned, the ear occupies a less prominent role than its other more central facial cousins such as the eye and the nose. Nevertheless, as those who suffer with them know well, prominent ears or *prominauris* can be a significant contributor to facial disharmony and unhappiness.

Many physicians are misled to believe that auricular surgery is easy. However, the achievement of perfect curvature of form and symmetry is as difficult today as when auricular surgery was first entertained and conceived some many hundreds of years ago. Dr. David Furnas, 30 years ago, said that surgery of the external ear was the one old-fashioned test for plastic surgeons, more than "sophisticated in-training examinations," and evaluations for re-certification, which "unfailingly separated the accomplished journeyman from the rest of the crowd, with grading of the test done by the studied glance of the common man" (Clinics in Plastic Surgery, July 1978). This statement was a testament to the astonishing intricacy of the auricle's form and to our collective specialties' sometime failings in realistically recreating that form that nature intended.

In today's modern age of surgery, the statement rings as true as the day it was made. While technology has allowed other facial plastic surgical techniques to surge forward in scope and outcome, cosmetic otoplasty continues to rely on time-tested techniques that are at the same time gracefully simple, yet exceedingly difficult to reproduce in a consistently reliable manner.

This volume will review the history of cosmetic Otoplasty along with aspects of anatomy, embryology, and clinical evaluation relevant to the remediation of specific deformities. Our preferred technique will be detailed alongside those of others with specific reference to applications for the most commonly encountered auricular abnormalities. The volume has been organized in an effort to provide an easy-to-follow, step-by-step approach to cosmetic Otoplasty taken from pre-operative considerations through post-operative management. We hope you find it useful to your practice.

Peter A. Adamson, MD, FRCSC, FACS
Jason A. Litner, MD, FRCSC

HISTORY AND PHILOSOPHY

PETER A. ADAMSON, MD, FRCSC, FACS AND
JASON A. LITNER, MD, FRCSC

Introduction

Reconstructive otoplasty techniques have been famously chronicled as far back as the 7th Century B.C. by the texts of Sushruta[1] and those of Tagliacozzi[2] in the 16th Century. In the modern age, the first report of otoplasty is attributed to a Prussian surgeon, Johann Friedrich Dieffenbach[3] who, in 1845, wrote of otoplasty in his seminal two-volume work "Die Operative Chirugie" that detailed reconstructive and general surgical methods of every type. In it, he described simple excision of skin from the postauricular sulcus with sutures affixing the auricle to the mastoid periosteum for the treatment of a posttraumatic auricular deformity. This was designed to set back the entire pinna with a tension closure.

The first purely cosmetic otoplasty technique was recorded by Ely[4], in 1881, who performed a full-thickness wedge excision of skin and cartilage to reduce a prominent auricle (**Figure 1-1**). Problems with this through-and-through skin and cartilage excision included noticeable anterior scarring and a sharp fold in the cartilage. Attempts to improve upon the technique by reduction in unacceptable scarring were advanced through to the 1890s by Haug, Keen, Monks, Joseph, Cocheril, Ballenger and Morestin[5,6]. All of these techniques, however, were reductive in nature and focused on excision of conchal skin and cartilage.

In 1910, Luckett[7] identified the unfurled antihelical fold as the cause for the classic lop-ear deformity as opposed to simple protrusion caused by an exaggerated auriculocephalic angle. This revelation

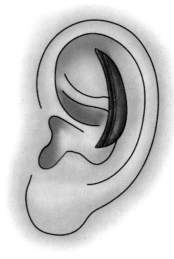

Figure 1-1. Ely's technique c. 1881. An anterior approach with full thickness crescentic excision of all layers for correction of the prominent ear.

permitted a focused procedure to 'recreate' the antihelix while leaving the anterior skin intact (**Figure 1-2**). A crescentic or fusiform excision of posterior skin and cartilage was undertaken in the proposed location of the antihelix. The scaphal and conchal cartilage edges created by this technique were plicated. Scarring was noticeably improved with this procedure, but a sharply demarcated cartilage ridge often could not be avoided.

Numerous modifications of Luckett's technique were soon to follow. In 1927, Alexander improved

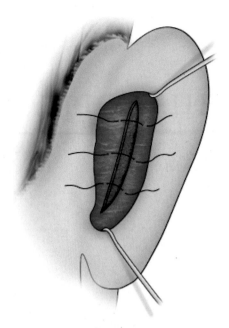

Figure 1-2. Luckett's technique c. 1910. Excision of a posterior strip of skin and cartilage along the desired antihelical line and plication with mattress sutures.

upon this technique by overlapping and suturing the cartilage edges in the high concha (**Figure 1-3**). In 1937, Davis and Kitlowski[8], pioneered the method of breaking cartilage spring via elliptical excisions of cartilage along the desired antihelical line, leaving intact "buttressing ridges" of cartilage to provide support. This was combined with stabilizing sutures and extensive postauricular skin excision to achieve a new antihelix. Sometimes, though, the postauricular sulcus was unnaturally obliterated

with this procedure. Young[9] reported a modification in which a more conservative postauricular skin excision was proposed along with excision of superior crus cartilage to prevent forward 'lopping' of the superior pole. Nevertheless, an unsightly step-off at the antihelical line remained with these methods.

The next significant advance is attributed to Becker[10] who, in 1949, described numerous cartilage excisions and incisions in an attempt to eliminate this unnatural ridging created by the earlier techniques and he used buried sutures to maintain these changes. Similarly, New and Erich used mattress sutures to maintain antihelical stability, but found that shaving or abrading the cartilage was just as adequate as excising whole fragments. Converse[11], in 1955, proposed a unique solution that eliminated the cartilage incision at the antihelical line to minimize the undesired ridging. Instead, parallel cuts were made isolating the antihelix via a posterior approach (**Figure 1-4**). Cartilage was then thinned with a wire brush, and tubed with suturing of the segments into elongated "cornucopias". Cartilage excision in the region of the concha was still advocated for treatment of excessive cupping. Additional contributions were made by Tanzer[12] in 1962.

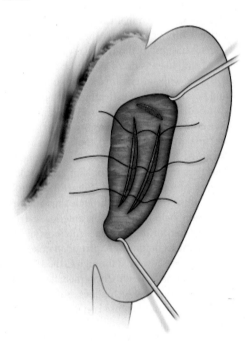

Figure 1-4. Converse's technique c. 1955. Slightly divergent incisions isolating the antihelix followed by thinning of the cartilage and tubing with mattress sutures.

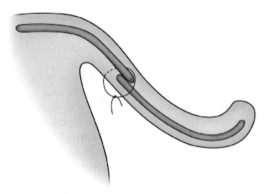

Figure 1-3. Alexander's technique c. 1928. Overlapping and fixation of the cut cartilage edges within the high concha.

Gibson and Davis[13], in 1958, demonstrated that relaxing incisions made in the perichondrium resulted consistently in bending of the cartilage in the opposite direction. Farrior[14] described a technique in 1959 that advised more judicious cartilage excision as compared to his predecessors, by excision of multiple longitudinal cartilage wedges to break cartilage spring before stabilizing the antihelix with suture. Stënstrom[15] described an otoplasty technique in 1963 that is still used by many today (**Figure 1-5**). This involved capitalizing on the tendency of cartilage to bend as noted by Gibson and Davis above. His was an anterior approach in which the lateral cartilage was scored or abraded to facilitate posterior bending via contraction of the intact posterior perichondrium. This technique was of particular utility in the setting of strong, stiff cartilage. However, it was frequently associated with anterior surface irregularities. Kaye[16] reported on his technique in 1967, which combined minimal-incision anterior scoring, posterior plication, and excision of a vertical ellipse of conchal cartilage.

Despite the varied and important contributions of the past century, incisional and excisional methods, dubbed cartilage-cutting otoplasty techniques, still presented a nagging problem, the tendency for unseemly anterior antihelical and conchal surface deformities. There was a distinct frameshift in evolution of the technique through the 1960s towards what has come to be known as cartilage-sparing methods, with the notable contributions of Mustarde[17] in 1963 and Furnas[18] in 1968. The emphasis

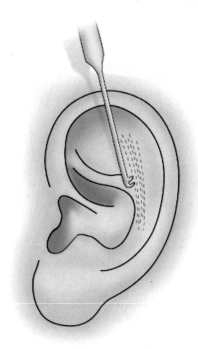

Figure 1-5. Stenström's technique c. 1963. Anterior subperichondrial scoring of the auricular cartilage at the proposed antihelical site using a specialized scratching instrument.

shifted for the first time from cartilage-cutting techniques to techniques that attempted to recreate the antihelical fold and set back the concha by use of suture alone (**Figure 1-6**). These approaches provided a more predictably natural auricular contour while eliminating displeasing anterior cartilage ridging.

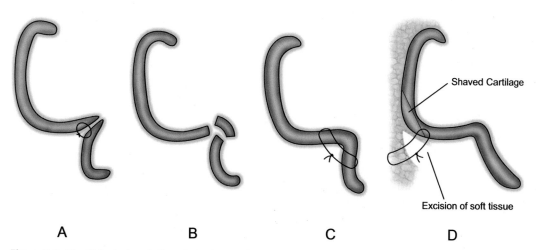

Figure 1-6. The historical evolution of otoplasty techniques from cartilage-splitting to cartilage-sparing methods. The technique of (A) Luckett, (B) Converse, (C) Mustardé, (D) Furnas and Webster.

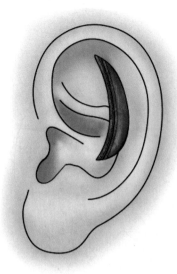

Figure 1-7. Mustardé's technique c. 1963. Recreation of the antihelix with three permanent transcartilaginous mattress sutures.

Mustarde, in 1963, described creation or redefinition of the antihelical relief using permanent transcartilaginous mattress sutures. Cartilage from the high conchal wall was 'borrowed' and rolled into the antihelix via scapha-conchal or scapha-fossa triangularis sutures, without the need for cartilaginous incisions and their associated surface irregularities **(Figure 1-7)**. In 1968, Furnas revived the concept of concha-mastoid sutures meant to address excessive vertical conchal height or cupping, originating from Gersuny's and Miller's early descriptions[19,20]. He further reported on additional suture methods[21] in 1978, including fossa triangularis-temporalis fascia sutures to medialize a protruding superior crus, and ear lobe-mastoid sutures to medialize a prominent cauda helicus.

These techniques were rapidly adopted because of the efficiencies they provided and the evident improvements. Webster[22] should best be credited with assimilation of all available techniques to provide a comprehensive approach to otoplasty, elements of which he practiced as early as 1952. His unifying technique effectively incorporated posterior skin and soft tissue excision, judicious conchal resection, anterior cartilage scoring, and antihelical mattress sutures. Additional sutures could be added as necessary. Further auricular 'set-back' could be achieved by tangential shaving at the depth of the conchal bowl cartilage, as previously described by Wright[23] in 1970.

To date, there are reported to be over 200 known otoplasty techniques. Most of these, however, represent slight modifications of the techniques previously listed in this chapter. Substantive additions relate more to means rather than methods, such as the novel use, by Raunig[24], of a diamond-coated file for anterior cartilage scoring. Fritsch[24] has popularized a novel incisionless otoplasty technique employing suture techniques via a transcutaneous approach.

Modern otoplasty technique places principal emphasis on achievement of a smooth, continuous auricular contour that is in proper relation to the cranium without the telltale sharp cartilage edges reminiscent of classical otoplasty results. In the next chapter, we will review aspects of external ear anatomy and embryology germane to the practice of cosmetic otoplasty.

References

1. Hauben DJ. Sushruta Samhita (Sushruta's Collection) (800–600 B.C.). Pioneers of Plastic Surgery. *Acta Chir Plast* 26:65, 1984.
2. Tagliacozzi G. De Curtorum Chirurgia per Institionem Libri Duo, *Venice*, 1597.
3. Dieffenbach JF. Die Operative Chirugie, Liepzig, F.A. Brockhaus, 1845.
4. Ely ET. An operation for prominence of the auricles. *Arch Ophthalmol Otolaryngol* 10:97, 1881.
5. Monks GH. Operations for correcting the deformity due to prominent ears. *Boston Med Surg J* 124:84, 1891.
6. Morestin H. De la reposition et du plissement cosmetiques du pavilion de l'oreille. *Revue Orthop* 4:289, 1903.
7. Luckett WH. A new operation for prominent ears based on the anatomy of the deformity. *Surg Gynecol Obstet* 10:635, 1910.
8. Davis JS, Kitlowski EA. Abnormal prominence of the ears: a method of readjustment surgery. *Surgery* 2:835, 1937.
9. Young F. Correction of the abnormally prominent ears. *Surg Gynecol Obstet* 78:451, 1944.
10. Becker OJ. Surgical correction of the abnormally protruding ears. *Arch Otolaryngol* 50:541, 1949.
11. Converse JM, Nigro A, Wilson FA, Johnson N. A technique for surgical correction of lop ears. *Plast Reconstr Surg* 15:411, 1955.
12. Tanzer RC. The correction of prominent ears. *Plast Reconstr Surg Transplant Bull* 30:236–46, 1962.
13. Gibson T, Davis WD. The distortion of autogenous cartilage grafts, its cause and prevention. *Br J Plast Surg* 10:257, 1958.
14. Farrior RT. A method of otoplasty. *Arch Otolaryngol* 69:400, 1959.

15. Stënstrom SJ. A natural technique for correction of congenital ear deformities. *Br J Plast Surg* 99:562, 1963.
16. Kaye BL. A simplified method for correcting the prominent ear. *Plast Reconst Surg* 52:184, 1967.
17. Mustarde JC. The correction of prominent ears using simple mattress sutures. *Br J Plast Surg* 16:170, 1963.
18. Furnas DW. Correction of prominent ears by conchamastoid sutures. *Plast Reconstr Surg* 42:189, 1968.
19. Gersuny R. Uber einige kosmetische Operationen. *Wien Med Wochenschr* 53:2253, 1903.
20. Miller C. Operations for correction of outstanding ears. In: Cosmetic Surgery. Philadelphia: *A.A. Davis;* 1925:201–11.
21. Furnas DW. Correction of prominent ears with multiple sutures. *Clin Plast Surg* 5:491, 1978.
22. Webster RC, Smith RC. otoplasty for prominent ears. In Goldwin RM, editor: Long-term results in plastic and reconstructive surgery. *Boston, Little Brown and Company,* 1980; p 146.
23. Wright WK. otoplasty goals and principles. *Arch Otolaryngol* 92:568, 1970.
24. Raunig H. Antihelix plasty without modeling sutures. *Arch Facial Plast Surg* 7(5):334, 2005.
25. Fritsch MH. Incisionless otoplasty. *Laryngoscope* 105:1, 1995.

2

ANATOMY AND EMBRYOLOGY

PETER A. ADAMSON, MD, FRCSC, FACS AND
JASON A. LITNER, MD, FRCSC

Introduction

Auricular protrusion may have some basis in evolutionary development because hearing can be demonstrably improved somewhat by cupping the ear or pulling it forward. While the concha is principally responsible for collecting sound waves and reflecting transmission into the external meatus, the auricular size and auriculocephalic angle also contribute to the acoustic resonance of the external ear[1]. Since much of our species no longer wanders the plains as a primary means of survival, the potential acoustic evolutionary fringe benefits of prominauris have ceased to be of importance. We are left only with its perceived aesthetic deficiencies or, at least, divergence from the 'norm'.

Auricular Histology

The external ear is composed of a thin, adherent anterior layer of skin and a thicker, loosely attached posterior cutaneous layer with a modicum of intervening subcutaneous areolar tissue on its posterior surface. This soft tissue envelops a single plate of dense connective tissue comprising elastic cartilage of 0.5 to 1 mm in thickness invested by perichondrium (**Figure 2-1**). Only the lobule contains no cartilage. It lies caudal to the cartilaginous scaffold and is composed of fibrofatty tissue. Also known as yellow cartilage, elastic cartilage is shared by the external auditory tube, the eustachian tube, and the supraglottic larynx. Like the more prevalent hyaline cartilage, type II collagen is a prominent feature of

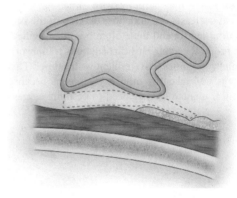

Figure 2-1. Cross-sectional view of the auricular cartilage demonstrating the relationship between cartilaginous framework and soft tissues.

its extracellular matrix but, in addition, it contains a dense network of delicately branched elastic fibers. This histologic distinction gives elastic cartilage its uniquely flexible properties.

While common in the developing body, cartilage is quite rare in the mature adult. Unlike other dense connective tissues, cartilage does not contain blood vessels or nerves, and depends on diffusion of nutrients for survival. Its extracellular matrix provides a powerful barrier to entry that makes it difficult, if not impossible, for antibodies and cells of the immune system to penetrate. The significance of these characteristics for facial plastic surgeons is that its low antigenic potential and slow metabolism makes cartilage, including that of the auricle, nearly perfectly suited for transplantation.

On the other hand, the chondrogenic activity of the perichondrium is limited to the period of active growth before the ear achieves full adult size. While matrix components can be produced throughout life, this production cannot keep pace with repair needs. If the cartilage is injured in adult life, the defect usually fills with fibrous tissue. A similar process arises when the cartilage is separated from its nutrient supply because of hematoma caused by trauma. This scenario affects the anterior cartilage contour exclusively, owing to the adherent nature of the perichondrium on the anterior surface of the ear. Although chondrogenic activity is minimal in this event, the fibrous tissue that arises within the intervening potential space can be quite dense. Along with this, scar contracture of the perichondrium itself may distort the auricular contour to produce the classic 'cauliflower ear' deformity.

Because of relatively poor access to nutrients, chondrocytes may atrophy with time. As water content decreases, small cavities develop in the surrounding matrix and these often become calcified. As a result, the adult ear's cartilaginous framework normally becomes less resilient with time. This point is well taken by otoplasty surgeons because technical maneuvers may need to be more aggressive in older patients in order to achieve and maintain the desired alterations.

Auricular Embryology

Embryology of the pinna is of greater interest to the reconstructive surgeon facing microtia repair. This is because the frequent coexistence of certain deformities of the pinna, acoustic canal, and middle ear structures may inform aspects of the planned repair. These elements are less informative with respect to cosmetic otoplasty but, nevertheless, they will be briefly reviewed.

The future ear makes its debut in the developing fetus in the third week of life with the emergence of the otic placode. The pinna itself is first apparent in week 6 of intrauterine existence as the hillocks of His[2], six primordial swellings or excrescences surrounding the dorsal surface of the first branchial groove. The three most cranial hillocks are attributed to the first branchial (mandibular) arch while the three most caudal hillocks belong to the second branchial (hyoid) arch.

Some controversy exists among embryologists as to what exactly happens from this point onward **(Figure 2-2)**. Professor His has contended that each

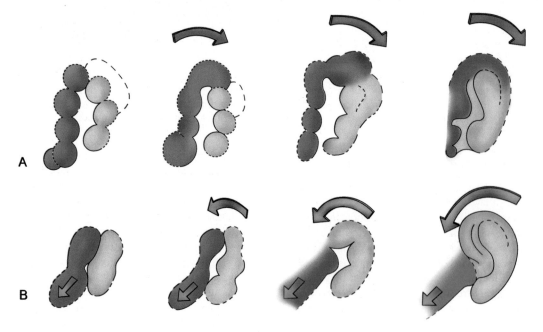

Figure 2-2. Theories of auricular embryology. (A) The theory of His in which the auricle is derived equally from the first and second branchial arches. Hillocks 1-3 are derived from the first branchial arch and hillocks 4-6 are derived from the second branchial arch. (B) The prevailing theory in which the first branchial arch contributes to the tragus and perhaps the helical root.

of hillocks 1-6 corresponds to a particular anatomic structure, namely, the tragus, the crus helicis, the helix, the antihelix, the antitragus, and the lobule, respectively. Schwalbe, conversely, has suggested that the helical margin emanates separately from a fold of skin adjacent to the hillocks and grows rapidly by the 12th week to overlie the underdeveloped antihelix[3]. Streeter[4], on the other hand, has deemphasized the hillocks entirely, contending that foci of mesenchymal proliferation are largely smoothed out by week 7 of development. Instead, the more rapidly growing hyoid arch mesenchyme increases its contribution to the pinna after week 8 to ultimately comprise 85% of the auricle. Only the tragus and, perhaps, the helical crus are derived from the mandibular first arch. This contention is supported by the anatomic location of congenital preauricular pits, which are located along a fusion plane at the intertragal incisure.

The concha, on the other hand, is thought to derive from the ectoderm of the first branchial groove. The upper portion forms the cymba concha, the mid-portion forms the cavum concha, and the lower portion forms the intertragal incisure. Failure of this aspect of auricular formation may lead to excessive lateral displacement of the pinna. Regardless of the specific derivations of the complex auricular structures, furling of the antihelix is thought to occur within the 12th to 16th weeks of development with furling of the helix occurring sometime

later during the sixth month of gestation. Failure of these processes to occur correctly will result in an overhanging or protruding scapha.

Abnormalities of mesenchymal proliferation leading to congenital deformities of the pinna may have strong genetic determinants. These can account for the striking familial patterns that are seen with some auricular deformities. In fact, Rhys and Bull[5] found 59% of patients affected by auricular abnormalities reported a positive family history. The transmission pattern was demonstrated by Potter[6] in at least one family to be of autosomal dominant inheritance with variable penetrance. This pattern of transmission can probably be extended to a majority of auricular abnormalities. Rogers[7] speculated that the entire spectrum of auricular deformities is, in fact, a continuum whose phenotypic severity rests on the degree of penetrance for the affected individual.

Auricular Anatomy

The cartilaginous framework of the auricle described above defines the intricate topographic highlights and lowlights that distinguish the external ear. The major landmarks are illustrated (**Figure 2-3 and 2-4**). Elevations on the visible lateral or anterior surface are met with corresponding depressions on the medial surface. The ear is bound to the skull over one-third of its medial surface with

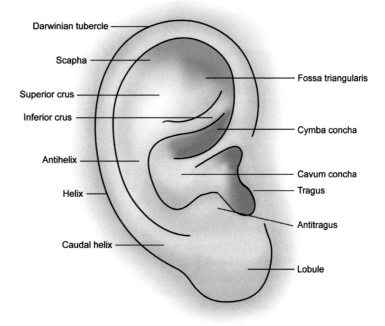

Figure 2-3. Anterior auricular surface topography.

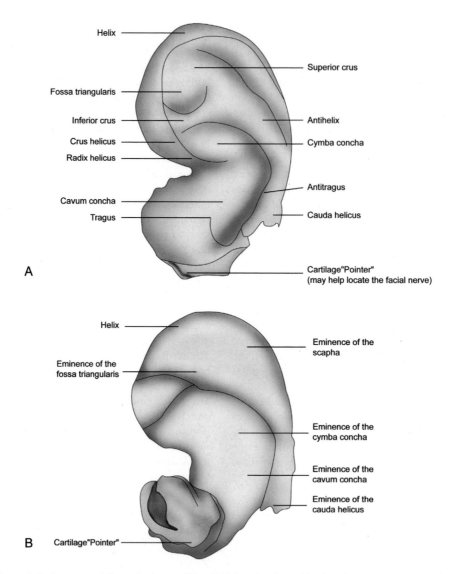

Figure 2-4. Anatomy of the auricular cartilage. (A) Anterior/lateral landmarks (B) Posterior/medial cartilaginous eminences.

the lateral two-thirds floating freely away from the skull. Major supporting ligaments preserve auricular stability. The anterior extrinsic ligament extends from the root of the zygomatic process to the tragus and helical spine, stabilizing the anterior auricle. Likewise, the posterior extrinsic ligament extends from the mastoid process to the posterior conchal wall, stabilizing the posterior auricle. Lastly, a third ligament passes from the tragus to the helix, bridging the cartilaginous external auditory canal. Additional supports are provided by the auricular

musculature and tightly bound skin. If the posterior ligament is underdeveloped or injured traumatically or surgically, the ear may be described as a 'flop' ear because of the obvious posterior auricular instability created.

There is a wide variation in normal auricular composition including the cartilaginous framework and lobular configuration (**Figure 2-5**). The cartilaginous framework may be arbitrarily divided into component subunits: the helix, the scapha, the concha, and the intertragal cartilage (**Figure 2-6**).

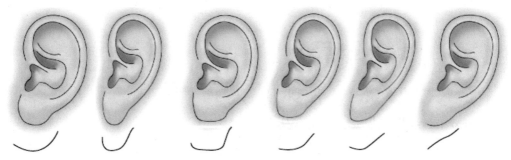

Figure 2-5. Variations in normal cartilaginous and lobular configuration.

The conchal bowl is separated into two distinct areas by the helical root, forming the cavum concha inferiorly and the cymba concha superiorly. The floor of the concha overlies the surface of the mastoid, whereas the vertical conchal wall stands perpendicular to the cranium. This relationship acts as a buttress to supply intrinsic support to the floating aspects of the auricle. The helical crus projects directly above the external meatus and extends upwards and backwards in a graceful arc that furls over its curvilinear descent to the cauda helicus and lobule. The antihelix endows a second arc, beginning at the antitragus and widening smoothly through its ascent and division into wider superior crus and a more sharply demarcated inferior crus. The fossa triangularis lies between the superior crus and the inferior crus of the antihelix and overlies the superior aspect of the temporal bone. The deep scaphoid fossa separates the helical rim and the superior aspect of the antihelical fold. A frequently observed cartilaginous protuberance along the lateral helical margin has been thought to correspond to a vestigial remnant of the tip of an animal's ear; this has been coined a Darwinian tubercle, although Darwin himself reportedly credited Woolner with this description[8].

The auricle receives sensory innervation from multiple sources **(Figure 2-7)**, including the 2nd and 3rd roots of the cervical plexus via the greater auricular (supplying much of the anterior auricle) and the lesser occipital nerves (supplying much of the posterior auricle). Lesser contributions are also made by the auriculotemporal nerve (V_3) supplying the anterior limb of the helix and the tragus, and the auricular branch of the vagus nerve (Arnold's nerve) which is also thought to carry some fibers from the facial nerve. Motor supply to the extrinsic auricular muscles arises from the temporal and posterior auricular branches of the facial nerve.

The vascular supply to the auricle comprises a robust network of anterior and posterior vessels **(Figure 2-8 and 2-9)**. Major arterial supply to the pinna arises from branches of the external carotid artery, including primarily the superficial temporal and posterior auricular arteries. A contribution is also made by a branch of the occipital artery. Venous drainage is analogous to the arterial supply, draining blood posteriorly to branches of the occipital and posterior auricular veins and anteriorly to the superficial temporal vein and on to the posterior facial vein. Lymphatic drainage is well developed in the form of anterior, posterior, and inferior auricular lymphatics that are directed to the superior cervical nodes.

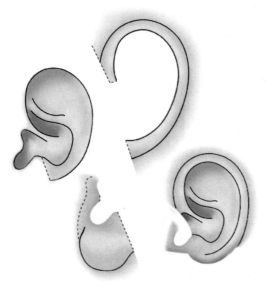

Figure 2-6. Aesthetic auricular cartilaginous subunits. The helical, scaphal, conchal, and intertragal components.

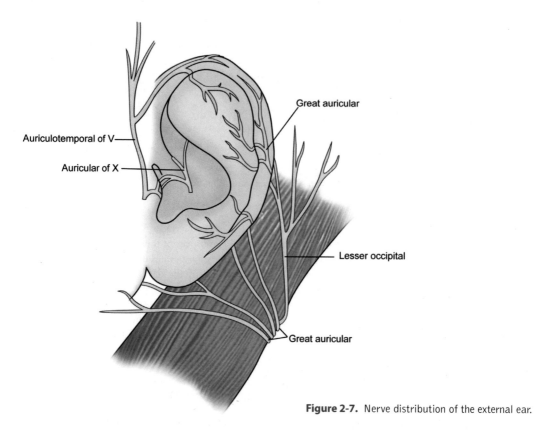

Figure 2-7. Nerve distribution of the external ear.

It appears that the vigorous auricular vascular supply is well matched to the metabolic needs of the cartilaginous superstructure in that disruption of one vessel will not generally compromise auricular viability. This composition has allowed for cartilage-cutting techniques of every variety to flourish without great concern for their effects. In the next chapter, we will review the aesthetic parameters of the cosmetically ideal ear along with specific deformities of interest to the otoplasty surgeon.

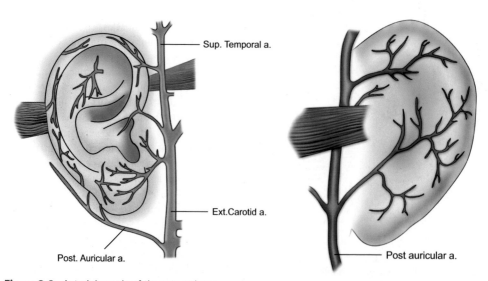

Figure 2-8. Arterial supply of the external ear.

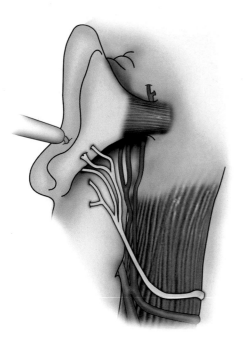

Figure 2-9. Nerve and venous distribution of the medial auricular surface.

References

1. Becker OJ. Surgical correction of the abnormally protruding ears. *Arch Otolaryngol* 50:541, 1949.
2. His W. Die formentwicklung des ausseren, Ohres. In: Anatomie menschlicher embryonen, Part III. *Leipzig: FCW Vogel,* 1985.
3. Schwalbe G. Die Ohrmuschel. Handbuck der Anatomie des menschem. Vol 5. *Jena: G Fischer,* 1987.
4. Streeter GL. Development of the auricle in the human embryo. *Contributions to Embryology* 14:111, 1922.
5. Rhys Evans PH, Bull TR. Correction of prominent ears using the buried suture technique: a ten year survey. Cited in: Rhys Evans PH. Prominent ears and their surgical correction. *J Laryngol Otolaryngol* 95:881, 1981.
6. Potter EL. A hereditary ear malformation transmitted through five generations. *J Hered* 28:255, 1937.
7. Rogers BO. Microtic, lop, cup and protruding ears: four directly inheritable deformities? *Plast Reconstr Surg* 41(3):208, 1968.
8. Webster RC, Smith RC. Otoplasty for prominent ears. In: Goldwin RM, ed. Long-term results in plastic and reconstructive surgery. *Boston: Little, Brown & Company,* p. 146, 1980.

3

AESTHETIC PARAMETERS AND SPECIFIC DEFORMITIES

PETER A. ADAMSON, MD, FRCSC, FACS AND
JASON A. LITNER, MD, FRCSC

Introduction

There is a wide variability among naturally appearing ears that would be considered to fit into the 'normal' range. One must first realize that interaural differences, sometimes significant ones, occur with some frequency. In one of the lead author's studies, asymmetries of scaphal size were noted in 15% of patients and differences in cephalic migration of the ears were noted in 11% of patients[1]. Nevertheless, a normal-appearing ear should fall within certain parameters. Normal relationships between auricular and facial proportions are depicted in **Figures 3-1 and 3-2**.

The distinction between normalcy and prominauris is quite literally a question of degree. The angle of greatest import is the auriculocephalic angle (**Figure 3-3**). This angle measures a tangent from the parietal scalp connecting a line that passes through the posterior-most position of the scapha. If one looks at standard deviation from the mean[2], one finds that 97% (two standard deviations) of ears have an auriculocephalic angle of between 25 and 35 degrees. Those exceeding this degree of angula-

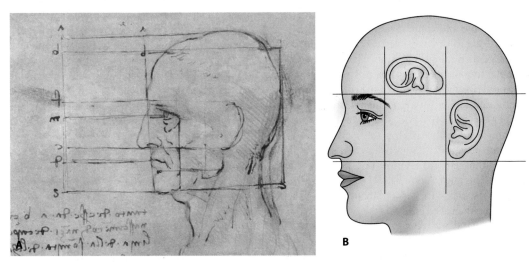

Figure 3-1. Auricular and facial proportions. (A) DaVinci's classical drawings of facial proportions indicating normal ear size and position. (B) The superior aspect of the proportionate ear is located on a vertical plane with the brow and is posteriorly inclined by approximately 20 degrees.

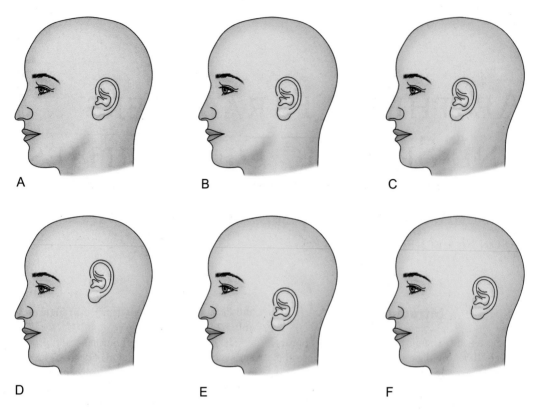

Figure 3-2. Correct auricular position. Only *A* is correctly positioned. *B* is too vertically oriented. *C* is too anterior. *D* is too high. *E* is too low. *F* is too posterior.

tion, and especially those exceeding 40 to 45 degrees, are usually regarded as abnormal, and the associated ears will appear to protrude.

The auriculocephalic angle may be deconstructed into two component angles, the cephaloconchal angle and the scaphaconchal angle. The cephaloconchal angle measures a tangent from the parietal scalp connecting a line that passes through the posterior-most position of the concha. This angle should ideally be greater than 45 degrees. The scapha-conchal angle has its vertex at the antihelix and measures a line passing through the posterior-most position of the concha connecting a line passing through the posterior-most position of the scapha. This angle should ideally be no greater than 90 degrees so that the fossa triangularis faces laterally rather than anteriorly.

The helical rim should project symmetrically about 10 to 12 mm from the scalp at the upper helix, slowly increasing along its downward trajectory to roughly 15 to 20 mm from the scalp at the cauda helicis. The point of maximal helical protrusion relative to the cranium is generally lo-

cated at a point intermediate between the superior pole and mid-auricle. If the auriculocephalic distance is surgically over-reduced to within 10 mm, the pinna can take on a "stuck-down" appearance. Ideally, the upper third of the helix should be visible on frontal view 2 to 5 mm laterally behind the antihelix[3]. The antihelix should not be, under any circumstances, the most laterally projecting structure on frontal view. The helical rim should follow a smooth curve to lie just lateral to, or behind, the antihelix at the lower pole. A relative protrusion of the middle third of the helical rim is aesthetically acceptable. Similarly, a slight protrusion of the lobule is permissible, although it should lie within the plane of the scapha. The position of the ear lobe is determined by the lateral projection of the antitragus and the cauda helicis.

Auricular Deformities

Prominauris is, by far, the most common auricular deformity, affecting approximately 5% of the Caucasian population[4]. In fact, it may be the most com-

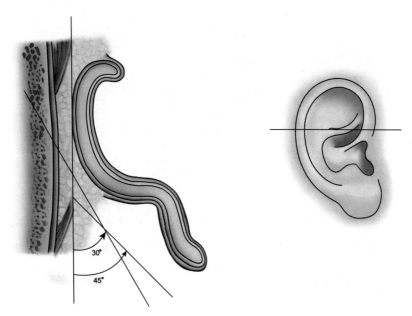

Figure 3-3. Auriculocephalic angle. An axial section showing an ideal auriculocephalic angle of about 30 degrees compared to a more obtuse angle observed when the antihelix is unfurled.

mon congenital deformity of the head and neck. This should be contrasted to congenital microtia, whose incidence approaches 1:20,000. It is important to note that other congenital abnormalities, predominantly those of the genitourinary tract, may coexist with these deformities.

Numerous pejorative and ignominious epithets have been foisted on auricular deformities, including: lop ear, cup ear, shell ear, Machiavellian ear, elfin ear, bat ear, elephant ear, Dumbo ear, butterfly ear, donkey ear, flop ear, jug ear, and more. All of the deformities of auricular shape can be distilled into a handful of causative features.

The most frequently noted abnormality is a relatively underdeveloped antihelix, especially at the upper pole along the superior crus. Most authors refer to this phenomenon as 'unfolding' or 'unfurling' of the antihelix. To the observer, this has the undesirable effect of allowing the contour of the concha to flow more or less directly into the scapha without any clear line of demarcation. The loss of auricular prominence in this region gives the appearance of flattening, lengthening, and consequent disproportion of the upper ear. Loss of acuity of the scaphaconchal angle leads to more anterior and lateral displacement of the upper helix and abnormal effacement of the fossa triangularis.

The second most frequently observed deformity is a misshapen conchal bowl with a high vertical con-

chal wall. Normally, the tragus and antitragus should project laterally about 1 cm from the depth of the conchal bowl. When the vertical conchal wall is abnormally high, the mid-portion of the helix will appear to protrude excessively. Holsen[5] attributed two thirds of cases of prominauris to an obtuse scaphaconchal angle and the remaining one-third to an oversized conchal wall. By contrast, in one of the lead author's studies, nearly 90% of patients displayed both conchal protrusion and antihelical unfurling[1].

A less common deformity is underdevelopment of the inferior crus of the antihelix, causing protrusion of the superior pole[3]. Likewise, a deficient helical roll such as in the eponymous Machiavellian ear, though less common, will cause a distinctive flattening of the auricular margin. Finally, protrusion of the ear lobule may aggravate the appearance of a prominent ear.

Specific Auricular Syndromes

The myriad of auricular forms may follow a continuum depending on the influence of genetic and teratogenic predeterminants at various times during embryogenesis. Nevertheless, a select few specific auricular syndromes that are pertinent to otoplasty can be characterized (**Figure 3-4**).

The *lop ear* is so-named because of its overly shortened appearance. This owes to the faulty

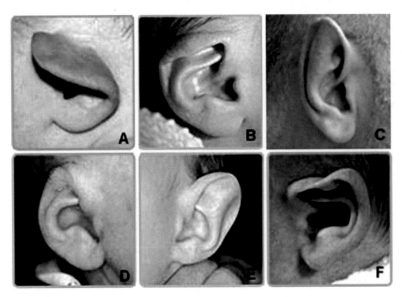

Figure 3-4. Various auricular deformities. (A) Prominent ear (B) Lop ear (C) Macrotia (D) Cryptotia (E) Stahl's ear (F) Kinked helical rim. (*Photos courtesy of Mr. David Gault, www.earreconstruction.co.uk.*)

maturation of the antihelix, scapha and, to some degree, the helix itself. As a direct result, the upper pole of the ear hangs limply, demonstrating an acute downward fold and appearing smaller than normal. This downward fold usually occurs at the auricular tubercle but may appear more medially, thereby eclipsing the anterolateral portion of the concha. Lopping of the pinna is often further exacerbated by the presence of poor cartilage resiliency.

The *protruding ear* is brought about by the unfurling of the antihelix, especially at its superior crus, often accompanied by excessive vertical conchal height or lateral angulation. Protrusion of the cauda helicis may require that the lobule be addressed as well. In general, the shape and size of the ear approaches that of normal auricular relationships and proportions.

The *cup ear* is aptly named because of its overdeveloped, deeply concave concha. This deformity creates an exaggerated concentrically cupped appearance to the upper pole, helix, and lobule, which may be coincidentally shortened. The entire vertical height of the ear may, accordingly, appear smaller than normal. The form of the cup ear therefore stands somewhere between that of the lop ear and protruding ear. Unlike the lop ear, however, the cartilage is often quite thick, rendering a lasting correction more difficult.

The *shell ear* derives its moniker from incomplete development and absence of furling of the helical rim. This can accompany an obtuse angle of the helical root as it abuts the scalp. The resultant shallow helical roll can give the upper and middle pole a flattened appearance typified by a half-shell.

The *satyr ear* or *elfin ear* draws its name from the characteristic pointed helical contour produced by incomplete furling. The tip of this misshapen helix is thought to correspond to the tip of an animal's ear as displayed in Greek mythology.

The *Machiavellian ear* is similar to the satyr ear, but it additionally entails a large, flattened scapha with typically thin cartilage. Rarely, this may be associated with complete macrotia, or an ear that is truly enlarged in all dimensions.

Finally, in *Stahl's ear*, an extraneous, posteriorly located, transversely oriented third antihelical crus is present. This is often combined with an underdeveloped superior crus and flat helical roll. Scaphal anomalies may also be present.

Although deformities are understandably manifold with an anatomic structure as richly complex as the external ear, the significance to the facial plastic surgeon is to be able to properly recognize those frequently associated abnormalities within each subunit of the auricle. This will allow the surgeon to predictably address each of these deficiencies without fear of omission. In the chapter to follow, we will review aspects of clinical assessment, surgical planning, and photographic documentation of otoplasty cases to allow for consistent sharing and comparison of results.

References

1. Adamson PA, McGraw BL, Tropper GJ. Otoplasty: critical review of clinical results. *Laryngoscope* 101(8):883, 1991.
2. Wodak E. Cited In: Minderjhan A, Huttl WR, Hildman H. Mustarde's otoplasty: evaluation of correlation between clinical and statistical findings. *J Maxillofac Surg* 8:241, 1980.
3. Wright WK. otoplasty goals and principles. *Arch Otolaryngol* 92:568, 1970.
4. Bardach J. Congenital ear deformities. In: Surgery for congenital and acquired malformations of the auricle. In: Cummings CW, Fredrickson JM, Hawker LA, Krause CJ, Schuller DE, eds. Otolaryngology Head and Neck Surgery. *St. Louis: CV Mosby,* p. 2861, 1986.
5. Holsen L, Vedung S. Reconstructing the antihelix of protruding ears by perichondrioplasty: a modified technique. *Plast Reconstr Surg* 65:753, 1980.

4

CLINICAL EVALUATION, SURGICAL GOALS AND PSYCHOLOGICAL IMPLICATIONS

PETER A. ADAMSON, MD, FRCSC, FACS AND
JASON A. LITNER, MD, FRCSC

Introduction

Otoplasty does not qualify as an extraordinarily common procedure. It is performed in approximately 15 per 100,000 people per year. Nevertheless, as with all facial plastic surgical procedures, otoplasty requires careful preoperative consideration and planning to achieve consistently favorable results. A surgeon's particular otoplasty practice will vary depending on practice location and demographics. In our practice[1], approximately two-thirds of cases are in the pediatric age group with approximately 50% of cases performed in patients between 5 and 9 years of age. The distribution of sexes slightly favors females by a ratio of 5:4. Peaks in demand for the procedure coincide with entry to school, adolescence, and early adulthood when psychological pressures reach their heights. As would be expected, secondary otoplasty is chiefly the province of adults.

As with any procedure, it is of paramount importance to elicit the patient's specific complaints about his or her ears. A secondary deformity noted by the surgeon, such as a prominent Darwinian tubercle, may be of little concern to the patient. The psychological impact of the perceived deformity should be explored and met with an empathic response. Clearly, young children will be unable to voice specific concerns, but they can express a general sense of distress imposed by this condition. Ensuring emotional as well as physical maturity is an essential component of the preoperative assessment. Historical features of interest in addition to general medical fitness are a personal or family history of bleeding tendencies, poor wound healing, and hypertrophic scarring or keloid formation. As mentioned in an earlier chapter, the genetic penetrance is variable, so one should inquire about other family members similarly affected.

Physical Examination

Each ear must be examined separately in relation to each other and to other facial features. Although both ears tend to be affected similarly, they can be so affected to varying degrees. A systematic approach to evaluation is advisable to reveal the precise anatomic features responsible for the observed deformity. This will mitigate against the potential neglect of coexistent deformities that might form a basis for surgical undercorrection. The data sheet (**Figure 4-1**) has proven a useful assessment tool in our practice. Overall symmetry of auricular size, contour, projection from the scalp, and proportion to other facial features should be noted with patient and/or parental attention called to any asymmetries. The auricle should measure 5 to 6 cm in vertical height and the long axis should recline about 20 degrees from the vertical plane. This is more or less parallel to the dorsal nasal contour. Additional secondary auricular measurements and angles are highlighted (**Figure 4-2**). Assess the helix for contour irregularities. The interrelationship between the auricular subunits (concha, helix, antihelix, and lobule) should be recorded. The presence of other craniofacial anomalies should also be documented.

Inadequate antihelical folding may occur throughout its course or at the superior or inferior crus alone. Isolated superior pole prominence may often result from an underdeveloped inferior crus[2]. Excessive prominence or unfurling of the helical rim may also be present. An excessively deep and high-walled conchal bowl should be identified, if present. The auricle is occasionally laterally displaced by a hyperpneumatized mastoid bone[3]. Less frequent deformities include an outstanding lobule or cauda helicis, prominent tragal or antitragal cartilage, or the presence of a Darwinian tubercle.

In addition to estimation of the auriculocephalic angle, cephaloconchal angle, and scaphaconchal angle described in the previous chapter, excursion of the helical rim should be routinely measured at three points corresponding to each vertical third of the auricle (**Figure 4-3**). These measurements should be taken in such a way as to be reliably reproduced, as follows:

1 The mastoid-helical distance at the most superior point along the helical rim
2 The mastoid-helical distance at the most laterally projecting point along the helical rim, usually at the level of the external auditory meatus
3 The mastoid-helical distance at the level of the intertragal incisura

Ideal measures for these points are roughly 10 to 12 mm superiorly, 16 to 18 mm in the middle third, and about 20 mm at the cauda helix. Consistency in these measurements allows for precise interaural comparisons (**Figure 4-4**). Additional measurements that may be advocated by some authors are the distance from the top of the helical rim to the

bifurcation point of the common crus, and measurement of the scaphal width. These measures can give the surgeon a sense of whether scaphal or helical shortening procedures might be helpful in restoring balanced proportions to the auricle.

The ear should then be palpated in two strategic locations. First, a cotton-tipped applicator may be utilized to apply posterior pressure to the conchal wall. Flattening and deprojection of the concha will allow the surgeon to estimate the degree of conchal setback, if any, that would be desirable. This procedure also permits an assessment of the amount of postauricular skin redundancy. Second, gentle medial digital pressure on the helical rim will allow for simulated accentuation of the antihelical fold to determine the extent of surgical correction required. As part of this manipulation, the pliability of the cartilage framework should be assessed, as this will directly inform the degree of requisite surgical cartilage weakening.

Photographic Assessment

As with any procedure, replicable photographs aid in conveying results to patients and colleagues. We find several standard views to be highly informative, including a frontal view, bilateral full-facial and close-up views, and a posterior view. Some surgeons also favor a bird's eye, craniocaudal photo that is particularly useful in demonstrating lateral auricular projection. An elastic headband may be necessary to help expose the ears. Care should be taken to respect the Frankfort horizontal plane. Postoperative photographs are typically repeated at six and twelve months postoperatively.

Surgical Goals

The foremost goal of otoplasty is the recreation of aesthetic parameters and proportions of the external ear that are at once symmetrical, intrinsically balanced with respect to individual auricular components, and extrinsically harmonious with other facial features. One should strive for pleasingly natural contours without surface irregularities, cartilaginous edges, or other indications of surgical intervention.

A set of utilitarian guidelines for the otoplastic surgeon has been put forth by McDowell[4], and elaborated upon by Mallen[5]. This is highlighted in **Table 4-1**. In order to achieve symmetry, a bilateral procedure is indicated in almost every

ADAMSON ASSOCIATES
COSMETIC FACIAL SURGERY
Otoplasty Assessment

Patient Name _____ Age _____

Assessment Date _____ O.R. Date _____

Case – Primary _____ Revision _____

Type of Deformity _____

Deformity	Right	Left	Treatment	Right	Left
Conchal Wall			Mastoid Soft Tissues Cartilage Shave		
Helix Protrusion			Concho-mastoid Suture Fossa-Fascia Suture		
Antihelix Unfurling			Scapho-Conchal Sutures		
Cartilage Strength			Scapho-Fossal Sutures Cartilage Scoring		
Lobe Protrusion			Reduction Plasty		
Scapha			Reduction Method		
Helix Deformity			Darwin's Tubercle Exc. Cartilage Scoring		
Cephalic Position Asymmetry			Correction Tension Suture		
Other			Skin Excision Skin Suture Type Cartilage Excision Other		

Measurements	Pre-op ↓	Post-op ↓ →			
Date	_____	_____	_____	_____	_____
Right Top Mid (Apex) Lobe	_____ _____ _____	_____ _____ _____	_____ _____ _____	_____ _____ _____	_____ _____ _____
Left Top Mid (Apex) Lobe	_____ _____ _____	_____ _____ _____	_____ _____ _____	_____ _____ _____	_____ _____ _____

Results	Right	Left

Subjective
  1. Patient
  2. Doctor
	_____
	_____
		_____
		_____

Objective (McDowells)
  1. No Protrusion upper 1/3
  2. Helix Visible to Mid Ear
  3. Helix Smooth
  4. Post-Auricular Sulcus
  5. Symmetry _____
	_____
	_____
	_____
	_____
	_____
		_____
		_____
		_____
		_____
		_____

Complications
1. Hematoma
2. Infection
3. Granuloma
4. Suture Spit
5. Scar hypertrophy/Keloid
6. Other

Unsatisfactory Result   Patient   /Doctor
1. Why
2. Recurrence
3. Other (explain)
4. Revision (Why?)

Figure 4-1. The data sheet used by the senior author (PAA) for both preoperative assessment and recording of operative measures.

case. Protrusion of the upper pole must be corrected and, only then, minor protrusion of the lower pole may be acceptable. Wright has indicated that medialization of the helical rim should ideally be undertaken to within 15 mm of the scalp[2], although we have found that adhering to the three measurements noted above yields highly satisfying outcomes. The antihelix should arc smoothly and gently from its origin upward to the superior crus, and it should not be excessively pinched or narrowed. The helical rim should be visible just lateral to the antihelix and antitragus on frontal view, at least down to the middle third of the auricle. The antitragus should be proportionately sized. The tubercle of Darwin, if present, should not be prominent. The postauricular sulcus must be maintained.

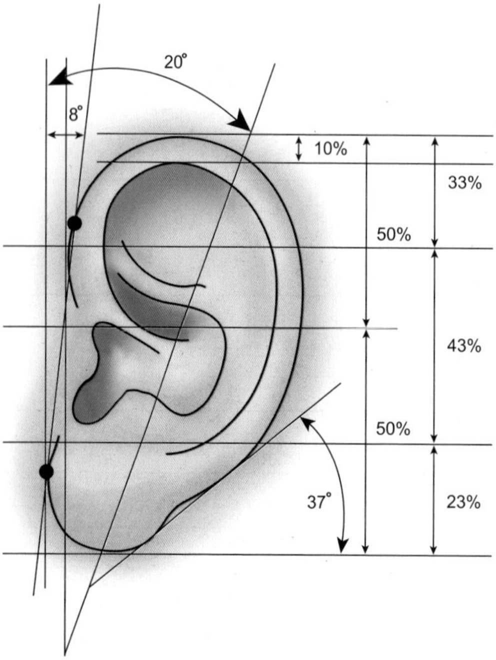

Figure 4-2. Various auricular angles and proportions of auricular subunits. Note the long axis of the ear of 20 degrees, the axis of the superior to inferior otobasion of 8 degrees.

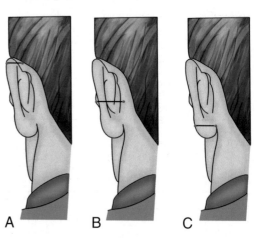

Figure 4-3. Auricular measurements according to anthropometric guidelines. (A) The superior auriculocephalic distance is measured from the mastoid to the most superior aspect of the helix. (B) The medial auriculocephalic distance is measured from the mastoid to the most lateral aspect of the mid-helix. (C) The inferior auriculocephalic distance is measured from the mastoid to the most lateral point of the helix at the intertragal incisure.

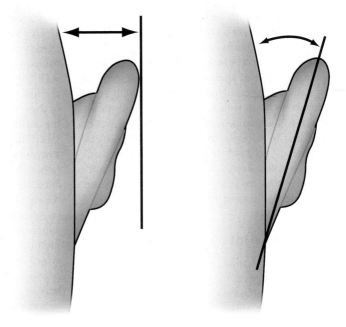

Figure 4-4. View from above of measurement of auricular angles and distances. Consistent measures can be difficult. Measurement of distances is easiest from the scalp to the most laterally projecting edge. Measurement of angles is best done along the axis of the auricle.

If these principles are observed, the chances for postoperative satisfaction are enhanced.

Psychological Implications and Timing of Surgery

Prominauris has been often said to be a sign of good fortune in the Far East; however, at least one surgeon we know of East Asian background has disputed

TABLE 4-1   Mcdowell's Goals of Otoplasty[4]

1. All trace of protrusion of the upper pole must be corrected. Some residual protrusion of the middle and lower thirds is acceptable providing the upper third is corrected. However, the reverse does not hold true.
2. From the frontal view, the helix should be seen lateral to the antihelix, at least down to the mid-auricle.
3. The helix should have a smooth and regular line throughout.
4. The postauricular sulcus should not be markedly decreased or distorted.
5. The ear should not be placed too close to the head. Auriculocephalic distances should measure 10–12 mm superiorly, 16–18 mm at the mid-auricle, and 20–22 mm inferiorly
6. Interaural comparison of auriculocephalic distances should be within 3 mm between ears at any given point.

this claim (Joseph Wong, MD, personal communication). Certainly, in western cultures, prominauris is often met with ridicule starting from an early age[6]. For unknown reasons, this deformity appears to inspire a unique propensity for derision among children. During these formative years, particularly ruthless taunting on the part of schoolmates or other peers can have a devastating impact on the fragile psyche of the developing child. Children affected by prominauris have been noted to react to such treatment with an inclination towards aggression and petulant behavior.

In one study of adolescents exhibiting problem behaviors, 40% were observed to have auricular deformities[7]. The corollary is true as well in that the incidence of psychological and behavioral disturbances has been found to be elevated in children with prominauris. In this age group, affected individuals do not have well-developed defense mechanisms, and these are easily overwhelmed to produce near constant feelings of insecurity, inadequacy, and anxiety neurosis[8]. Children affected by low self-esteem typically respond by withdrawal and introversion or by engaging in problem behavior. The harmful impact of these feelings may expand to influence social development and academic performance. In fact, many affected young patients have reported academic setbacks as a result of this ill-treatment[9].

Adults are not immune to this type of prejudice as well. Adults with prominauris have been maligned through their perceived association by others with negative characteristics such as dishonesty, stupidity, and even criminality[10]. This type of prejudgment may conspire against the social or professional aspirations of affected individuals. As a result, some adolescents and young adults are paradoxically driven to overcompensate and excel in athletics or academia in response to their perceived cosmetic handicap. A majority of adults, nevertheless, continue to suffer from varying degrees of insecurity and may seek for years to disguise their auricular deformities with camouflaging hairstyles.

Nonsurgical Intervention

Ideally, surgery could be avoided entirely for auricular prominence. The practice of noninvasive auricular splinting in the neonatal period is frequently applied in Japan. The idea behind this practice is that sustained pressure may guide the growth and shaping of the pliable auricular cartilage during infancy, at least for deformational auricular anomalies (see Figure 4-5). This stands in contrast to malformational anomalies in which normal chondrocutaneous auricular components are deficient.

Various splinting methods have been employed, including surgical tapes, conforming bandages, tissue adhesives, dental splints, and thermoplastic splint materials among others. It was once thought that the effectiveness of these techniques was limited to the early neonatal period up to 6 months of age. Matsuo et al.,[11] reported differential responses with cases of Lop ear and Stahl's ear responding only to immediate nonsurgical correction while protruding ears responded until about 6 months of age. This technique was also effective for cryptotia, a condition in which the superior pole is often covered by a fold of skin and is lacking in lateral projection.

Of interest, the same authors[11] reported an extremely high rate of auricular deformities in Japanese babies, occurring in as many as 55% of neonates, with 84% of these spontaneously disappearing in the first year of life. By the age of 1, the incidence of these deformities approached 5 to 7%, similar to the incidence noted in the Caucasian population. Protruding ears appeared to increase significantly in frequency by 1 year of age, suggesting an acquired rather than a congenital mechanism. They postulated that recurrent turning of the baby's head folded the ear forward, resulting in an acquired protrusion.

Subsequent studies[12] have reported that sustained nonsurgical splint application over several months was successful in remodeling auricular growth in a majority of Japanese patients older than one year of age and up to age 14. Similar studies[13,14] have extended the benefits of early intervention to Western populations but have failed to reproduce demonstrable improvement for infants splinted after 3 months of age, although there has been a recent suggestion of success in splintage programmes for children as old as 18 months (personal communication, Mr. David Gault). Thus, for those children who have passed beyond the neonatal period, surgical intervention appears to be the only reliably permanent method for correction of prominent ears.

Timing of Surgery

The age at which otoplasty is undertaken is decidedly important as it is one of the few elective plastic surgical procedures carried out in children. Thus, the burden of choice often falls to the parents to ascertain what will secure their child's best future interests. Some parents may be fraught with indecision while others may advocate intervention for

Before

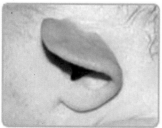

During

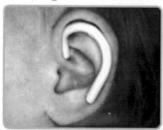

After

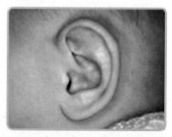

Figure 4-5. An example of an external molding device for splinting of the prominent ear. (Photos courtesy of Mr. David Gault, www.earbuddies.co.uk.)

their children whom have not yet achieved psychological readiness. The surgeon must account for the psychosocial dynamics of the entire family when planning surgery in the pediatric population.

The fact that the potentially damaging emotional consequences of prominauris appear to escalate with time argues for early corrective surgery. Very young children may not perceive a problem with their ears. School age children tend to grow appreciably in self-awareness levels and may begin to suffer the earliest consequences of mockery. The surgical experience for the family is far more positive when the child is keenly interested and cooperative in the process rather than reluctantly following along. So, an opportune time for intervention would appear to be prior to this transition point around age 5 or 6. However, other factors such as auricular growth must be considered in determining the optimal timing for otoplasty.

At 1 year of age, the ear has reached about 80% of its adult size, measuring 5 cm in vertical height on average compared to 6 cm for the adult ear[15]. By age three, 85% of auricular growth has been attained[16]. Steady growth continues to occur over the first years of life to near completion by age 5 or 6[17]. Ear width and distance from the scalp change very little after age 10. Continued elongation of the lobule may give the illusory appearance of continued auricular growth with age though this is more than likely solely the effect of gravity.

Some surgeons suggest that otoplasty may even be performed from the age of 3 because most affected ears are already larger than normal[15]. However, most surgeons recommend that surgery be performed in the year before the child begins schooling. Prior to the age of 5 or 6, there is some theoretical concern that surgery might impede additional auricular growth. After this age, the risks of potential growth hindrance are substantially diminished. For this reason, we prefer to delay surgery until the child is 5 or older. If the child's auricles appear smaller than normal, we may postpone the procedure until the age of 6 or 7.

Of final influence is the quality and pliability of the auricular cartilage. The auricular cartilage in youth is characteristically compliant. With passing years, cartilage resilience diminishes and, with it, the probabilities of a lasting correction in the absence of more extreme cartilage manipulation.

Therefore, earlier intervention favors both potentially greater realization of the psychological benefits of otoplasty and facilitation of the procedure with greater technical ease. In the next section, we will feature step-by-step detailed descriptions of our preferred graduated cartilage-sparing otoplasty technique in addition to those of other experienced otoplasty surgeons.

References

1. Adamson PA, McGraw BL, Tropper GJ. Otoplasty: critical review of clinical results. *Laryngoscope* 101(8): 883, 1991.
2. Wright WK. Otoplasty goals and principles. *Arch Otolaryngol* 92:568, 1970.
3. Minderjahn A, Huttl WR, Hildman H. Mustarde's otoplasty: evaluation of correlation between clinical and statistical findings. *J Maxillofac Surg* 8:241, 1980.
4. McDowell AJ. Goals in otoplasty for protruding ears. *Plast Reconstr Surg* 41(1):17, 1968.
5. Mallen RW. Otoplasty. *Can J Otolaryngol* 3(1):74, 1974.
6. Tanzer RC. Congenital deformities: deformities of the auricle. In: Converse JM, ed. Reconstructive Plastic Surgery, 2nd ed. *Philadelphia: WB Saunders,* 1977.
7. Adamson JE, Horton CE, Crawford HH. The growth pattern of the external ear. *Plast Reconstr Surg* 36:466, 1965.
8. Becker OJ. Surgical correction of the abnormally protruding ears. *Arch Otolaryngol* 50:541, 1949.
9. Rhys Evans PH, Bull TR. Correction of prominent ears using the buried suture technique: a ten year survey (unpublished). Cited in: Rhys Evans PH. Prominent ears and their surgical correction. *J Laryngol Otol* 95(9):9881, 1981.
10. Rogers B. Microtic, lop, cup, and protruding ears. *Plast Reconstr Surg* 41:208, 1968.
11. Matsuo K, Hayashi R, Kiyono M, Hirose T, Netsu Y. Nonsurgical correction of congenital auricular deformities. *Clin Plast Surg* 17(2):383, 1990.
12. Yotsuyanagi T, Yokoi K, Urushidate S, Sawada Y. Nonsurgical correction of congenital auricular deformities in children older than early neonates. *Plast Reconstr Surg* 101(4):907, 1998.
13. Tan ST, Abramson DL, MacDonald DM, Mulliken JB. Molding therapy for infants with deformational auricular anomalies. *Ann Plast Surg* 38(3):263, 1997.
14. Tan S, Wright A, Hemphill A, Ashton K, Evans J. Correction of deformational auricular anomalies by moulding – results of a fast-track service. *N Z Med J* 116(1181):U584, 2003.
15. Mallen RW. Otoplasty. *Can J Otolaryngol* 3(1):74, 1974.
16. Maniglia AJ, Maniglia JV. Congenital lop ear deformity. *Otolaryngol Clin North Am* 14:83, 1981.
17. Adamson JE, Horton CE, Crawford HH. The growth pattern of the external ear. *Plast Reconstr Surg* 36: 466, 1965.

5

Marking, Infiltration, and Soft Tissue Management

Peter A. Adamson, MD, FRCSC, FACS and
Jason A. Litner, MD, FRCSC

Introduction

The available techniques for surgical correction of prominauris will generally fall along one or more of the following surgical avenues:

1. Excision of skin and perichondrium with a tension closure
2. Cartilage excision techniques
3. Cartilage incision techniques aimed at breaking cartilage internal 'spring' (these may include morselization, scoring, abrading, scratching, etc.)
4. Excision of soft tissue with or without tangential shave of the conchal floor cartilage to permit conchal setback
5. Suture techniques to 'splint' or maneuver the auricular framework into a more favorable anatomic relationship (these include incisionless suture techniques)

The techniques broadly categorized above are listed in order of descending levels of surgical aggressiveness. Thus, a suture maneuver, on balance, is less aggressive and, therefore, less likely to result in a permanent deformity than, say, a maneuver further up the list, such as a cartilage-cutting technique. For this reason, we prefer cartilage-sparing techniques wherever possible with cutting techniques reserved

for only those situations where they are deemed warranted.

To consistently achieve favorable outcomes, we proceed with otoplasty in a systematic and graduated stepwise fashion via a postauricular approach. Our approach is predicated on a thorough preoperative and intraoperative assessment of each deformity present so that a specific individualized surgical plan can be properly devised and implemented. This approach entails a logical progression, beginning with variable amounts of postauricular skin and soft tissue excision. Cartilage management consists of conchal setback followed by antihelical contouring always in the stated order, with cautious assessment and correction of each deformity along the way. The cauda helicis is then addressed in the setting of lobe protrusion while the fossa triangularis is addressed in the setting of persistent superior pole protrusion. Finally, any requisite ancillary procedures such as lobule, helical, and scaphal reductions are undertaken.

Intraoperative overcorrection is not only necessary but is, in fact, critical to long-term satisfaction, as postoperative recovery of elastic recoil will result in loss of as much as 40% of correction[1,2]. Undercorrection is normally interpreted by patients as a surgical failure and, so, slight overcorrection is to be preferred over the alternative. Provisions taken in anticipation of such elastic recoil of the auricular cartilage, particularly at the superior pole, will often avert an unsatisfying outcome. Even in the setting of a unilateral deformity, bilateral surgery is often advisable because corresponding forces of recoil should act equivalently on both ears to result in a symmetrical postoperative outcome. As a rule, the most affected ear is operated upon first as any final minor adjustments towards the conclusion of the procedure are made easier when later dealing with the least affected ear.

Surgical Technique

Preparation and Incision

Most patients and surgeons, at least for surgery within the pediatric population, favor general anesthesia for cosmetic otoplasty, but some may choose local anesthesia with intravenous sedation for this procedure. The latter type of anesthesia is quite well tolerated in the adolescent and adult population. An effective drug 'cocktail' for adults of average size includes 10 mg of morphine and 50 mg of dimenhydrinate or their equivalents given 1 hour preoperatively. This is followed by 6 mg of diazepam administered intravenously just before infiltration of local anesthe-

sia with additional 2 mg increments provided as needed to titrate for comfort. We also pretreat with 1 g of cefazolin and 125 mg methylprednisolone or their equivalents to preclude possible complications. Proportional doses by weight are given in children. Individual anesthesiologists, if utilized, will each have their own favored drug protocol.

A conservative amount of hair is trimmed in the postauricular area. One-inch sterilizing tape is placed circumferentially around the head just behind the hairline to keep stray hairs out of the operative field. Both ears are prepped and draped simultaneously into the field with 1% chlorhexidine aqueous solution to allow interaural comparisons to be readily made intraoperatively. Prior to local infiltration and associated tissue distortion, the area of redundant postauricular skin to be excised is estimated by gentle posterior manipulation of the ear with traction in the desired position (**Figure 5-1**).

Postauricular Skin Excision

In earlier otoplasty techniques, the skin excision was typically centered over the medial aspect of the desired antihelical fold. Perichondrium was often included in this excision. As we know, bending of the antihelix will occur at its greatest line of weakness. Following the principle of the lever arm, the

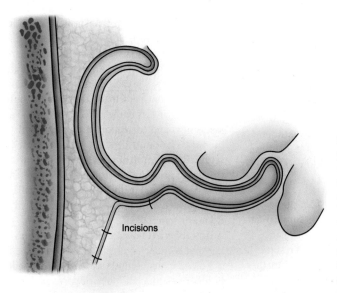

Incisions

Figure 5-1. Planning of the postauricular incision by posterior manipulation of the auricle in order to estimate the degree of skin and soft tissue excess. This cross-section shows that the planned incision should be eccentrically placed falling more on the posterior concha rather than over the mastoid. This will ensure that the incision does not lateralize onto the postauricular skin and become visible.

closer the cutaneous defect is to the helix, the greater will its furling action will be on the antihelix. If the incision is based over the desired antihelical line, much of the medialized cartilage tension is easily transferred to the soft tissue along the line of closure. As a result, an unacceptably high incidence of wound complications, suture extrusions, and hypertrophic scarring can be noted.

Therefore, our excision is designed and marked with eccentric placement over the postauricular sulcus with greater extension onto the posterior concha than onto the mastoid (**Figure 5-2**). In this way, forces acting on the medialized cartilage are distanced from the soft tissue closure. In addition, as the ear is set closer to the head, the final scar will tend to lie in the preserved postauricular sulcus rather than behind it as may happen in the frequent event of posterior scar migration. Lastly, this eccentric placement facilitates better cartilage exposure and placement of sutures. The apices of the excision are maintained at least 1 cm from the superior and

inferior poles so that the resultant scar will be concealed from view.

The auricular and mastoid soft tissues are then extensively infiltrated with a solution of equal parts 1% lidocaine with 1:100,000 epinephrine and 0.5% bupivacaine with 1:200,000 epinephrine to aid in vasoconstriction and hydrodissection. The bupivacaine allows for some slightly longer acting anesthesia to aid in a smooth and painless postoperative transition. Typically, from 5 to 10 mL of this mixture will be sufficient to secure adequate vasoconstriction and anesthesia. When placed in the plane just superficial to the perichondrium of the posterior scapha, it also provides some hydrodissection.

The lateral limb of the incision is then taken down to the auricular perichondrium. The medial limb of the incision is taken down to the mastoid periosteum and temporal fascia. The skin excision is then accomplished in continuity with variable amounts of mastoid soft tissues (i.e., fat and postauricular muscle) down to periosteum to permit the desired degree of conchal retrodisplacement (**Figures 5-3 and 5-4**). The depth of the soft tissue excision will depend on the prominence of the conchae cymba and cavum. Little to no soft tissue excision is necessary inferior to the level of the antitragus. Usually, the fusiform area of skin excision is about 10 to 12 mm at its widest point.

Soft Tissue Management

The posterior auricular skin is then widely undermined and a superolateral releasing incision may be undertaken at this juncture to facilitate suture placement in the area of the upper pole and fossa triangularis. Specifically, placement of scapha-fossa and fossa-fascial sutures is greatly facilitated through this releasing incision. Hemostasis is meticulously maintained throughout this process with bipolar electrocautery.

Intraoperative photos of our preferred skin and soft tissue management in otoplasty are shown in **Figure 5-5**. While cartilage overcorrection is preferred to undercorrection, this is not so with respect to the degree of postauricular skin excision. Overly enthusiastic skin excision will not make for better correction. On the contrary, aggressive skin and soft tissue resection is given to possible blunting and obliteration of the postauricular sulcus with development of a "stuck down" appearance that is most unappealing. Likewise, closure of the skin under tension is similarly to be avoided for fear of widening and hypertrophy of the scar.

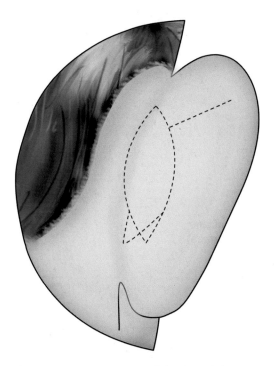

Figure 5-2. A posterior view of the planned skin excision. The excision is fusiform in shape and may be extended inferiorly in an open book manner to aid in medialization of a protrusive lobule. A superolateral releasing incision is completed to gain greater access to the superior pole cartilage.

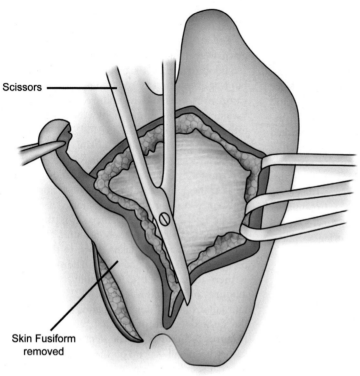

Scissors

Skin Fusiform
removed

Figure 5-3. The skin and soft tissue excision is accomplished in continuity down to the level of the auricular perichondrium, the mastoid periosteum, and the temporalis fascia to allow for adequate conchal setback.

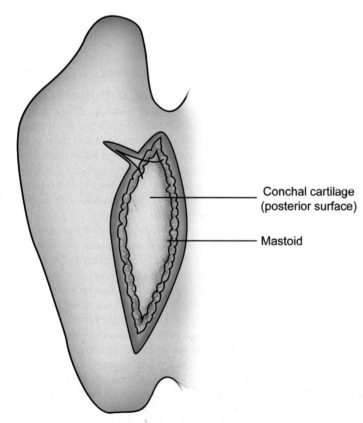

Conchal cartilage
(posterior surface)

Mastoid

Figure 5-4. The auricle at rest at the conclusion of the skin and soft tissue excision. Note that the auricular perichondrium and mastoid periosteum are skeletonized. The excision should overlie the posterior concha without compromising the postauricular sulcus.

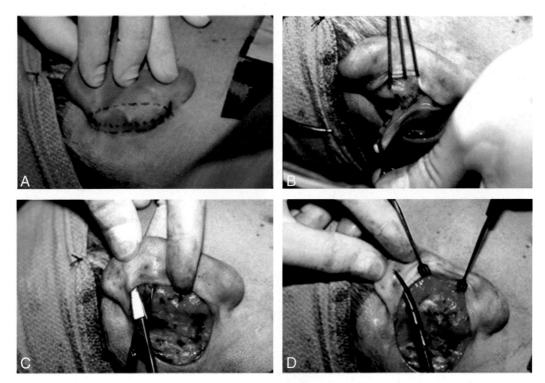

Figure 5-5. Intraoperative photos showing the sequence of skin and soft tissue excision. (A) Planning of fusiform skin excision so that it maintains the natural postauricular sulcus. (B) Excision of skin and soft tissues in continuity down to the auricular perichondrium and mastoid periosteum. (C) Wide undermining of the postauricular skin to the helical margin in a supraperichondrial plane, and (D) Performance of a superolateral releasing incision to better allow for scaphaconchal suture placement.

As in a face lifting procedure, the correction is maintained by cartilage manipulation so that there need be no tension on the skin closure. With this end in mind, Woolf and Broadbent[3] astutely recommend excision of postauricular skin at the termination of the case, limiting this excision only to the evident redundant skin. This is especially useful for the novice otoplasty surgeon, as he or she need not feel the pressure of judging correctly at the outset of the operation. We have found, however, that the skin excision may be accomplished at the beginning of the case if one is assiduous and precise about estimation of skin and conchal excess. In this way, postoperative scar widening can be avoided. Other authors[4,5] have suggested unique skin incisions for the very same purpose such as the double-spindle incision preferred by Hinderer for avoidance of a postoperative telephone ear deformity (**Figure 5-6**).

In select cases in which an excessively large conchal bowl or hyperpneumatized mastoid is contrib-uting to lateralization of the auricle, preparation can be made to affect a greater degree of medialization by wider excision of the mastoid soft tissues. Such undermining will aid in repositioning and retrodisplacement of the auricle. However, it must not be carried out more extensively than 5 to 10 mm posterior to the external auditory meatus, for fear of losing auricular support and ensuing impingement on the meatus. Further to this end, tangential shave of the conchal bowl, release of auricular cartilage attachments, or drilling of the mastoid is rarely needed to achieve the desired degree of medialization.

We must reiterate that the skin and soft tissue excision comprise the least amount of skin necessary to eliminate redundancy and to permit appropriate setback of the concha with a tension-free closure. In the next chapter, we will describe our cartilage-sparing approach for management of the cartilage to achieve a lasting and natural-appearing correction of the prominent ear.

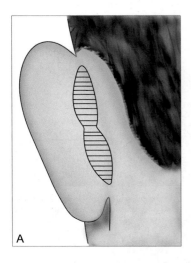

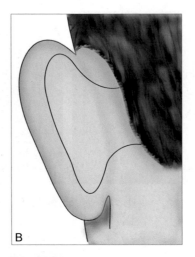

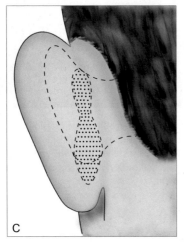

Figure 5-6. Alternative skin incisions and excisions. (A) Dumbbell excision designed to prevent a postoperative 'telephone ear' deformity (B) Medially based postauricular flap with excision reserved for the end of the procedure, and (C) Inclusion of a lobule-correcting inferior skin excision with either of the above excisions.

References

1. Adamson PA, McGraw BL, Tropper GJ. Otoplasty: critical review of clinical results. *Laryngoscope* 101(8): 883, 1991.
2. Adamson PA, Kraus WM, Strecker HD. Aesthetic Otoplasty. In: Willet JM, editor. Facial Plastic Surgery. Norwalk, CT: *Appleton and Lange* 1997; p 331.
3. Woolf RM, Broadbent TR. Repositioning of prominent ears. *Ann Plast Surg* 1(2):154, 1978.
4. Hinderer UT, Del Rio JL, Frenegal FJ. Otoplasty for prominent ears. *Aesth Plast Surg* 11:63, 1987.
5. Mallen RW. Otoplasty. *Can J Otolaryngol* 3(1):74, 1974.

6

Cartilage Management

Peter A. Adamson, MD, FRCSC, FACS and
Jason A. Litner, MD, FRCSC

Introduction

Cartilage-sparing techniques involve suture manipulation of the prominent auricle to achieve and maintain a normal anatomic contour and position. The use of isolated suture techniques is appropriate when the auricular cartilage is still pliable enough to maintain correction by suture alone. We find that most patients up to young adulthood will fall into this category. The surgeon must appreciate the cartilage consistency to determine the need for additional cartilage-weakening procedures. Patients with less resilient cartilage may yet be amenable to suture correction but may require supplementary maneuvers in the form of cartilage scoring or shaving to increase the probability of a permanent improvement. We undertake management of the cartilage in the prominent ear using a graduated approach, relying primarily on suture techniques while reserving more aggressive handling of the cartilage for those cases that are unlikely to respond favorably to suture techniques alone.

The hallmark of suture methods in otoplasty is respect for the integrity of the cartilaginous auricular framework. Suture techniques possess numerous distinct advantages over cartilage-cutting approaches. These include:

1. Great versatility of correction based on nearly unlimited possibilities for differential placement of sutures
2. Maximal preservation of cartilage integrity with minimal cartilage injury, scarring, or destabilization
3. Relative ease of execution to achieve surgical correction
4. Control of final intraoperative refinement to achieve interaural symmetry by simple suture adjustment
5. Avoidance of possible long-term auricular surface pebbling or irregularities
6. Finally, potential for reversibility

Since the initial descriptions of these suture techniques, countless combinations and modifications have been advanced[1-6]. The advantageous features highlighted above have permitted these techniques to revolutionize otoplastic surgery. Unlike with cartilage-cutting maneuvers, there is no point from which the surgeon may not return. Positioning of the suture(s) may be trialed out and altered as desired without fear of consequences in the form of permanent injury to the cartilage. Correction may be precisely controlled at multiple levels prior to final tightening of the knots. For these reasons, we utilize cartilage suture techniques via our own graduated approach as the workhorse of our otoplasty method.

Suture methods may be broadly categorized according to specific anatomic placements and their intended uses. Scaphaconchal sutures may create an antihelical fold where one does not exist, or they may be called upon to accentuate or modify an existing antihelical fold. Scapha-fossa triangularis sutures will allow a similar outcome to be effected on the superior crus. Fossa triangularis-temporalis fascia sutures are invoked in order to draw the auricular framework, along its superior aspect, closer to the head. A comparable result may be produced for the lower aspect of the cartilaginous framework utilizing conchamastoid sutures. Finally, a protuberant lobule may be medialized via caudaconchal sutures or subcutaneous lobule-sternomastoid muscle sutures. These same sutures may be manipulated to modify the vertical angulation of the ear and to displace the ear in cephalad or caudad directions.

Surgical Technique

Conchal Setback

The amount of soft tissue excision to be performed deep within the postauricular sulcus depends on the degree of conchal setback desired, for it is this excision that allows the conchal cartilage to be retropositioned. As discussed in the previous chapter, appropriate soft tissue excision is critical to the achievement of acceptable conchal cartilage setback via a suture medialization technique. Conchal setback is particularly helpful for those prominent ears in which a high conchal wall is a major component of the deformity and, in fact, normalcy of auricular position cannot be achieved in these cases without aggressive conchal management. In most cases, relatively more soft tissue is excised superiorly than inferiorly, as this is where a greater correction of protrusion is required.

We find it most logical to proceed firstly with setting the appropriate vertical position and angulation of the concha relative to the head, and secondarily adjusting the antihelix in relation to the fixed conchal position. Many authors consider the underdeveloped antihelix to be the primary abnormality present in the prominent ear, and they so choose to correct this deformity initially. Too often, we find, proceeding in this order is imprudent, as it will risk antihelical overcorrection (especially in the region of the superior crus) and conchal undercorrection, with possible development of a postoperative "reverse telephone ear" deformity. Following conchal setback via our preferred graduated method, one may commonly find the necessary degree of antihelical manipulation to be less than previously thought or even, at times, completely unnecessary.

We typically make use of three Furnas-type horizontal mattress sutures of 4-0 Mersilene to secure the concha to the soft tissues and mastoid periosteum overlying the lateral skull, once the soft tissue deep to the conchal bowl has been excised[4] (**Figure 6-1**). The advantage of a braided, synthetic, nonabsorbable polyester suture material such as Mersilene (polyethylene terephthalate) is its ease of handling, permanence, and general tissue tolerability. The braided nature of this particular suture permits accurate correction and secure knot tying with precise tension, and without much risk of postoperative stretch. However, this braided nature may also be impugned for its ability to colonize bacteria, adding slightly to infection risk and, with it, the threat

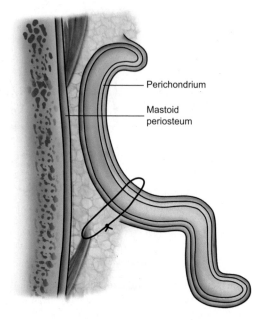

Figure 6-1. Conchamastoid sutures secure the conchal bowl to the mastoid periosteum and include both lateral and medial perichondrium and intervening cartilage, but not anterior skin. The vector of pull should entail posterior traction.

of suture rejection and extrusion. For this reason, a monofilament permanent suture such as Prolene (polypropylene) provides a suitable alternative, though one must then contend with the potential for stretch and decreased knot stability over time. Whatever suture material is chosen for correction, it is notable that it should be of light color so that it does not show through the anterior skin postoperatively.

The tension involved in mobilization of the auricular cartilage is borne initially by suture stabilization and subsequently by the inflammatory tissue response around the areas where sutures were placed. The sutures form and splint the cartilage into its new position until some permanence is derived from a binding scar tissue reaction, generally over the first several weeks to months after surgery. For this reason, some authors may choose a long-acting dissolvable suture such as Vicryl (polyglactin 910) rather than a permanent suture[7]. Absorbable sutures or PDS (polydioxanone) alleviate the risk of long-term suture extrusion but may elicit a greater inflammatory response during the initial healing phase that may bring into play other hazards such as poor wound healing. Theoretically, the fibrotic tissue that is ultimately laid down is sufficient to maintain repositioning with remodeling of the auricular cartilage. However, the inherent spring of mature auricular cartilage in older teens and adults may lead to stretching of the scar tissue with time and eventual recurrent protrusion. For this reason, we favor use of a permanent suture correction at this time for all of our suture otoplasty techniques.

Of great importamce to the graduated approach is the particular sequence in which these sutures are placed. The first suture is placed in the superior-most aspect of the floor of the fossa triangularis and through the mastoid periosteum. It is clamped and left untied until the remaining sutures are placed. With this suture, the bowl is drawn posteriorly and superiorly so that the compressed conchal cartilage does not unwittingly encroach upon the external auditory canal. A full thickness bite is taken, consisting of posterior and anterior perichondrium and intervening cartilage, but not skin. Anterior palpation of the bowl skin with the finger pad or fingernail is inordinately helpful to ensure suitably deep suture placement. While it is important that the suture engage the anterior perichondrium laterally, it is equally important that the mastoid periosteum be engaged medially to prevent suture slippage and pull-through. The needle should have a solid feel when the bite is taken. The trial sutures should be pulled under some tension prior to tying down to test them for durability and slippage.

Second and third sutures are placed along the identical vectors in the inferior bowl (cavum concha) and mid-bowl (cymba concha), respectively, drawing the conchal cartilage posteriorly and superiorly. A substantial bite of mastoid periosteum is taken to ensure adequate long-term suture stability. Once all sutures are appropriately positioned, they are tightened in the same order in which they were thrown. In this way, the mid-bowl can be adjusted to align with the superior and inferior aspects. This aids in the prevention of overzealous tightening within the mid-bowl region and a resultant "telephone ear" deformity. Only once final suture adjustments have been made are all of the knots fully tightened down to achieve a final correction.

We have found several points of critical importance in avoiding potential complications related to this technique (**Figure 6-2**). The *superior* vector of pull on the concha is essential to minimize infringement on the ear canal. Similar conchal distortion or external auditory canal compression may occur by too high placement of a suture on the conchal wall with subsequent anterior displacement of the bowl.

Overtightening of the conchal sutures, particularly within the mid-bowl, is to be expressly avoided. The vector of pull is significant not only with respect to medial displacement but also with regard to angulation and vertical positioning of the ear. Depending on the particular placement of sutures in concert with soft tissue dissection, the auricular position may be influenced in both a vertical plane and in terms of cephalic-caudal angulation. Slight overcorrection of all sutures is preferred to allow for some cut-through; however, this should be accomplished uniformly. Relative overcorrection within the middle one-third of the ear is highly discouraged, as this will predispose to a "telephone ear" deformity, especially if the sulcal soft tissues have been over-resected.

If the conchal bowl is rather prominent, the mattress sutures may be placed higher up on the conchal wall to produce greater effacement of the bowl as the sutures are tightened. However, they must not be placed so high that they distort or rotate the bowl forward to compress the ear canal. This is especially true of the middle concha-mastoid suture, which, if located too far up on the wall of the bowl, may tend towards increased cupping and a "telephone ear" deformity. In addition, it should be recognized that, as the vertical height of the conchal wall is decreased by suturing the concha, the area of the horizontal floor of the concha is being proportionately increased. The ideal aesthetic should be sought with suture placement.

Rarely, even aggressive suture management of a prominent conchal bowl fails to achieve adequate medialization. The most likely explanation for such an unlikely scenario is one in which the posterior conchal eminences are overdeveloped. In this case, the overdeveloped cartilage will not allow acceptable posterior displacement by suture methods alone, as these contact points are preventing medialization because of their contact with the mastoid. In such cases, we find it advisable to reduce the excessively deep conchal bowl by tangential shave excisions of the ponticulus, triangular, and conchal eminences with a No. 10 or No. 11 blade. The extent and depth of conchal shave to be undertaken is dictated by the degree of overdevelopment (**Figure 6-3**). In extreme cases, a full thickness shave excision can be performed, but the anterior or lateral skin must be respected and preserved. This technique is preferred to anterior skin excisions or cartilage-cutting maneuvers, which can leave laterally visible scars and cartilage irregularities. Although seldom required, this maneuver can be very effective in

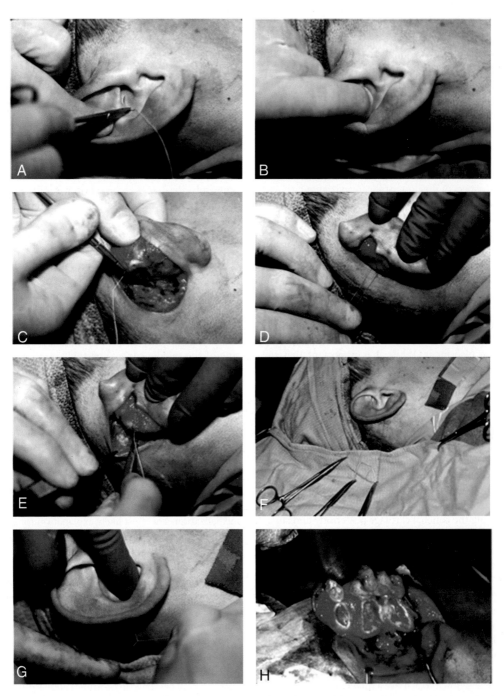

Figure 6-2. Intraoperative photos indicating the sequence of conchamastoid suture placement. (A) Posterior manipulation of the concha to decide on suture location. (B) Palpation of the concha with fingernail, providing tactile feel to prevent too superficial a 'bite.' (C) Placement of the first arm of the horizontal mattress suture while palpating the lateral surface. (D) Posterior vector of pull of the concha to decide on location of the mastoid suture. (E) Placement of the mastoid 'bite' to pull the concha posteriorly. (F) All sutures are clamped prior to tying down. (G) Sutures are thrown and tied in order of superior, inferior, and middle sutures while posterior traction is placed on the concha during suture tightening, and (H) Tangential shave of posterior cartilage eminences if greater conchal setback is desired.

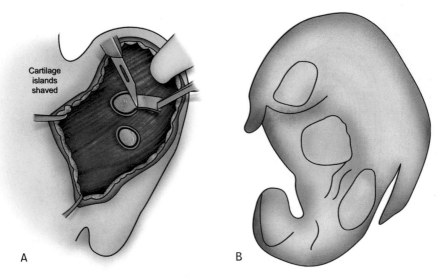

A   B

Figure 6-3. Cartilage island shaving for treatment of a persistently deep conchal bowl. (A) Shaving of cartilage using a No. 10 or 11 blade with preservation of anterior perichondrium. (B) Final view of shaved ponticulus, triangular, and conchal eminences.

allowing the concha to be further retrodisplaced into the surgically deepened sulcus (**Figure 6-2H**).

Antihelix Repositioning

We next turn our attention to the misshapen or absent antihelix. When appropriate conchal position is set, we often find a less than originally anticipated need for antihelical correction. Treatment of the antihelix is via two to four precisely placed 4-0 Mersilene Mustardé-type horizontal mattress sutures to recreate the antihelical furl (**Figure 6-4**). Again, the suture should transfix the full thickness of the cartilage and anterior perichondrium without impinging on, or tethering, the overlying lateral skin (**Figure 6-5**). Exposure of the peripheral reaches of the auricular cartilage for placement of the superior-most sutures may be enhanced by performance of a releasing incision or back-cut as detailed in the previous chapter. Engagement of the anterior perichondrium is critical to prevent suture pull-through. However, if the stitch is placed too superficially, engaging the dermis of the anterior auricular skin, then ulceration at the insertion site may result.

While some surgeons advocate use of ink, temporary sutures, or needle fixation to guide suture placement, we do not find these tools any more advantageous than careful digital palpation. Placement of such external devices, to our minds, unnecessarily contributes to soft tissue trauma. Under our protocol, the desired correction is manually

simulated as the surgeon applies external pressure using his fingernail at the preferred site on the anterior auricular surface. The surgeon can then

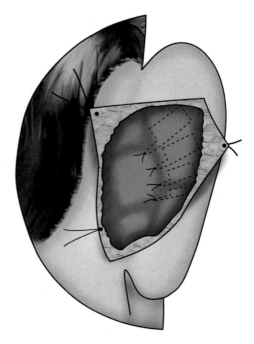

Figure 6-4. Posterior view of Mustardé-type scaphaconchal sutures to recreate the antihelical fold. The number of sutures required to create a smooth curvature varies from two to four.

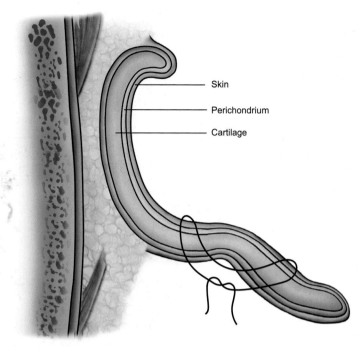

Skin

Perichondrium

Cartilage

Figure 6-5. Scaphaconchal sutures secure the scaphoid fossa cartilage to the vertical conchal wall cartilage. Sutures should engage medial and lateral perichondrium, but not anterior skin. Slight overcorrection is advised to allow for postoperative pull-through.

position the suture accordingly through palpation of this external pressure. The 'bites' of scaphaconchal sutures should be substantial enough to avoid cartilage pull-through, but not so large as to inadvertently cause buckling of the cartilage. Ideally, 'bites' of about 4 to 6 mm are more than adequate.

As with the conchal setback, a specific sequence is applied, whereby the superior and inferior crura are set as the initial maneuvers (**Figure 6-6**). We find that setting the superior-most and inferior-most sutures first creates 'jumping-off points' for construction of a gradually-arcing smooth curvature along the intervening antihelical ridge. By contrast, setting the suture first at the mid-portion of the antihelix may risk creation of an unnatural notch in this region because of overtightening or improper suture location.

The superior suture should extend from the superior-most scapha to the fossa triangularis. The inferior scaphaconchal suture is then placed at the most inferior portion of the antihelix between the inferior scapha and the highest portion of the conchal bowl. Finally, intervening sutures are variably and obliquely placed as needed to achieve a natural and continuous curvature of the mid-portion of the antihelical fold. The 'roll' of the antihelix should steadily thin out in width traveling in an antero-inferior direction. Judicious and accurate

suture placement and tightening is needed to generate a smoothly rounded curvature rather than a constricted antihelix or a conspicuous "post-like" appearance. As with our conchal setback technique, all sutures are first placed and then tightened in the same sequence to achieve the desired correction.

Many authors follow the teachings of Bull and Mustarde[8], who advocate placement of a prescribed number of sutures at equal distances from each other, usually about 2 mm apart. The suggested distance between limbs of each suture is approximately 1 cm while the ideal distance between outer and inner cartilage bites is 16 mm. This distance allows creation of a suitable curvature without notching or bunching of the intervening cartilage. Sutures that are placed too closely together risk overtightening with resultant weakening and notching of the cartilage, and creation of an unnatural curvature. Sutures that are placed too far apart or too close to the helical margin risk bunching of the intervening cartilage and creation of an antihelix of insufficient curvature, a so-called 'vertical post' deformity. Additionally, suture pull-through is a greater future risk since the suture tension is inadequately distributed.

The protocol stipulating a discrete number of equidistantly placed sutures may aid in achieving symmetric suture placement in both ears.

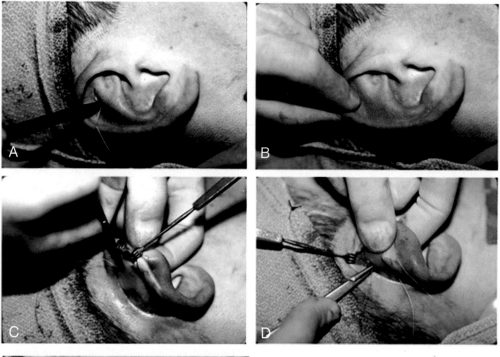

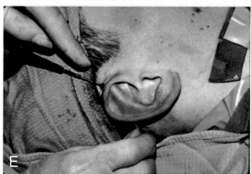

Figure 6-6. Intraoperative photos indicating the sequence of scaphaconchal suture placement. (A) Posterior manipulation of the scapha to decide on suture location. (B) Palpation of the scapha with fingernail, providing tactile feel to prevent too superficial a 'bite.' (C) Placement of the first arm of the horizontal mattress suture while palpating the lateral surface. (D) Placement of the conchal 'bite.' (E) Sutures are thrown and tied down in order of superior, inferior, and middle sutures once all sutures are appropriately placed; slight overcorrection is advisable.

As we know, though, both ears are not often symmetrical. We find it optimal, instead, to customize suture placement to achieve maximal contour advantage while minimizing chances for development of a "vertical post" deformity. To achieve the most natural curvature, suture placement should be concentric with respect to the center of the concha. In other words, the distance between the superior aspects of each mattress suture should be greater than the respective distance between the inferior aspects of each suture so that the suture line follows the intended arc of the antihelix.

The highest point of the antihelical roll will be produced along a line that is central between the superior location of the suture on the scapha and the inferior location of the suture on the concha. Eccentric placement of one or more sutures can be manipulated to effect the angulation of the new antihelix. This technique can be helpful when addressing a high conchal wall. If the conchal contribution to the prominent ear is relatively minor, it is possible to correct this by 'rolling' the excess conchal height into the antihelix when the scaphaconchal sutures are placed. This can be done by locating the conchal aspect of the mattress sutures further from the existing antihelix than is the scaphal part.

Once the conchal and antihelical positions are set bilaterally, measurements are once again performed at the three reference points used preoperatively to ensure symmetrical corrections. Target auriculo-cephalic distances at the mid-auricle are roughly 15 to 18 mm from the head in the intraoperative period. The final knot tying is then accomplished in the same order in which the knots were placed. Tying down the middle third sutures last discourages overtightening and resultant development of a "telephone ear" deformity. A small amount of overcorrection is desirable to mitigate future stretching and unfurling. The superior crus suture, especially, should be slightly overcorrected in a relative sense since this area is most likely to experience loss of correction. Of note, however, if the sutures are correctly placed in both number and location, then tension should be well enough distributed to the extent that significant overcorrection is unwarranted. Sutures in the middle third of the antihelix should not be overcorrected. Of importance, the antihelical sutures must not be tightened so much that the helical margin is drawn medial to the antihelical fold. The helix should always lie lateral to the antihelix on frontal view.

Mustardé has stressed the importance of knot placement in helping to create the desired antihelical contour[3]. He has advocated locating the knots inferiorly for the inferiorly placed sutures and superiorly for the superiorly placed sutures. His belief is that this knot placement will aid in pulling the cartilage into the correct shape.

Also of consequence is the positioning of the antihelical sutures with respect to the soft tissues. As the knots are tightened, the ear should be returned to its normal anatomic position and inspected with regard to the skin and soft tissues. One must be careful to position the sutures in such a way as to prevent a "bowstring effect" of the suture on the postauricular skin at the incision line. This effect bodes poorly for wound healing, promoting wound breakdown, granuloma formation, latent infection, and late suture extrusion.

Supplementary Maneuvers

Additional sutures may be placed as necessary to correct any remaining deformities (**Figure 6-7**). A persistently cupped superior pole may be addressed by added suture placement between the fossa triangularis and the temporalis fascia. In a review of 62 consecutive otoplasty patients from the senior author's (PAA) practice, only eight patients (13%) required fossa-fascial sutures[9]. Likewise, an equivalent prominence of the inferior pole may be remedied by suturing the cauda helicis to the mastoid. This maneuver was required in six patients (9.7%) in the same review[9]. Lobular protrusion is occasionally improved by placing a single cauda-conchal anchoring horizontal mattress suture.

We rarely resort to scoring or rasping of cartilage, although this is sometimes prudent in the extraordinarily stiff adult ear, wherein the anterior antihelical surface may be scored to encourage folding. This is done via tunnel access beneath the anterior perichondrium. We believe posterior cartilage

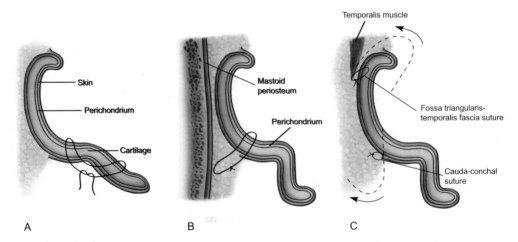

Figure 6-7. Summary of suture techniques in otoplasty. (A) Scapha-conchal sutures. (B) Concha-mastoid sutures, and (C) Fossa triangularis-temporalis fascia sutures and cauda-conchal sutures.

scoring to be contraindicated as it predisposes to further antihelical unfurling. In the previously cited review of the senior author's (PAA) otoplasty practice, only three of 62 patients required conchal cartilage shaving to achieve acceptable correction[9]. Whenever in question, we find it best to avoid such maneuvers as they are disposed to postoperative surface irregularities. However, the reverse argument is that cartilage weakening in the extraordinarily stiff ear will increase flexibility, facilitate furling, and reduce tension on the mattress sutures. For this reason, in the next section, we will highlight a number of techniques preferred by other authors that have a greater cartilage-weakening component.

In this chapter, we have reviewed management of the conchal and antihelical cartilage to achieve a stable and lasting correction of the prominent ear. These techniques have worked predictably for us in our otoplasty practice. In the next chapter, we will outline our preferred techniques for adjuvant correction of other associated auricular abnormalities, including a prominent lobule, an overdeveloped scapha, and an unfurled helix.

References

1. Morestin H. De la reposition et du plissement cosmetiques du pavillon de l'oreille. *Revue Orthop* 4:289, 1903.
2. Mustarde JC. The correction of prominent ears using simple mattress sutures. *Br J Plast Surg* 16:170, 1963.
3. Mustarde JC. Correction of prominent ears using buried mattress sutures. *Clin Plast Surg* 5(3):459, 1978.
4. Furnas DW. Correction of prominent ears with multiple sutures. *Clin Plast Surg* 5(3):491, 1978.
5. Rees TD, Wood-Smith D. Complications and untoward results. In: Rees TD, Wood-Smith D, eds. Cosmetic Facial Surgery. *Philadelphia: WB Saunders*, 1973; p. 556.
6. Webster RC, Smith RC. Otoplasty for prominent ears. In: Goldwin RM, ed. Long-term results in plastic and reconstructive surgery. *Boston: Little, Brown & Company* 1980; p. 146.
7. Riggs BM. Suture material in otoplasty. *Plast Reconstr Surg* 63:409–10, 1979.
8. Bull TR, Mustarde JC. Mustarde technique in otoplasty. *Fac Plast Surg* 2(2):101, 1985.
9. Adamson PA, McGraw BL, and Tropper GJ. Otoplasty: critical review of clinical results. *Laryngoscope* 101(8): 883, 1991.

Adjunctive Procedures: Management of the Helix, Scapha, and Lobule

Peter A. Adamson, MD, FRCSC, FACS and
Jason A. Litner, MD, FRCSC

Introduction

An enlarged concha and unfurled antihelix are the two major acknowledged contributors to the appearance of a prominent auricle. However, for a share of patients, a large scapha, unfurled helix, or an outstanding or enlarged lobule may distort auricular symmetry and further detract from an aesthetically acceptable auricular contour. These abnormalities may be corrected simultaneously with improvement of antihelical and conchal deformities to restore a naturally pleasing appearance to the ear. These refinements are generally performed as the final step in otoplasty, once conchal setback and antihelixplasty have been satisfactorily achieved. They may, however, be carried out independently, as they often are during otoplasty revision procedures.

Surgical Technique

Helical and Scaphal Abnormalities

Reduction of Helical Prominences

The principal helical abnormality encountered is the presence of a protuberant cartilaginous spine at the free margin of the helical rim, known as a Darwin's tubercle. It earned its moniker because this phenomenon is noted to be a feature or vestige of more primitive auricles. Most often, this occurs in combination with a well-formed helical margin. Remediation of a Darwinian tubercle is easily approached via a direct incision camouflaged at the lateral curl of the helix (**Figure 7-1**). Fusiform excision of a small portion of redundant skin is often performed to aid in re-drapage. A long rather than a short incision is preferred as this will facilitate skin closure without a standing tissue cone deformity. Incision is made under the helical fold to allow dissection up over the helical rim. The prominent barb of cartilage is excised and the incision is closed with a 6-0 nylon suture in a simple running fashion. Skin is trimmed from the upper flap to allow adequate draping over the helical rim. The resultant scar falls quite favorably along the line of the lateral helical curl.

On occasion, the helical rim is deficient and poorly developed, without the tight furl usually present in the normally formed auricle. This often occurs in conjunction with a prominent, abnormally high scapha, which, together with unfolding of the helix, produces an angulated helical rim that is often referred to as a 'Spock ear'. At times, this deformity is aggravated by a cartilaginous prominence of the outer helical rim. This cartilage may be shaved

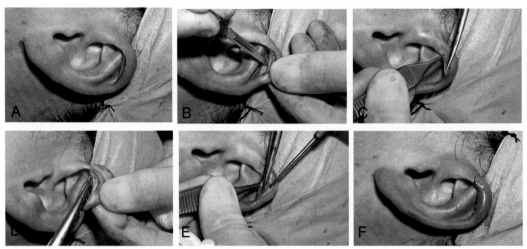

Figure 7-1. Intraoperative photos showing the sequence of excision of a Darwinian tubercle. (A) Marking of a fusiform skin excision that is slightly smaller than the planned cartilage excision. (B) Sharp skin incision. (C) Sharp resection of soft tissues with tissue scissors (D) Undermining with exposure of the cartilaginous tubercle. (E) Sharp excision of the involved cartilage, and (F) Skin closure without tension with a running nylon suture.

after a fusiform excision is made directly over the prominence. Excess skin is trimmed and closed after undermining.

Rarely, reduction of a prominent antitragus may need to be undertaken to achieve a balanced auricle. This can be accomplished with an anterior skin incision or with dissection along the antitragico-helicine fissure. Planning of the skin incision should bear in mind the potential for visible sequelae in this area.

Amelioration of a Deficient Helical Fold

The effaced helical rim can be treated in a manner comparable to the unfurled antihelix via the same posterior auricular incision. The posterosuperior releasing incision previously described in the context of soft tissue management is exceedingly useful in this endeavor. The postauricular skin should be widely undermined to the level of the helical rim and just onto the lateral surface of the auricle. Unlike with antihelical shaping, in order to obtain the desired effect, it is often necessary to slightly weaken the cartilaginous spring of the unfurled helix by scoring of its lateral aspect. Additionally, partial thickness incisions along the posterior surface of the helical rim may encourage anterior helical furling via the Gibson effect[1], wherein the cartilage tends to bend towards the side of intact perichondrium. This correction is secured by placement of a temporary through-and-through bolster to the involved area for 7 days.

If there is adequate cartilage stock, then this scoring maneuver may be all that is required to obtain the desired roll. On the other hand, if the cartilage is weak, further shaping may need to be undertaken by radial placement of scapha-helical mattress sutures along the involved extent of the helical arc. This is required to avoid cartilage instability. For the most severe deficiencies, the helical rim may be recreated by use of full-thickness helical wedge excisions (**Figure 7-2**). Alternatively, a cartilage graft may be utilized for this purpose. In this case, adequate skin coverage must be fashioned from the posterior skin flap. This flap may be advanced over the posterior scapha and doubled onto itself overlying the proposed new helical rim. A buried resorbable suture may coapt the two opposing dermal surfaces. The donor area of the medial scapha is left to heal secondarily if small, or it may be covered with a full thickness postauricular skin graft if large.

Reduction of a Large Scapha

If the auricular circumference is abnormally large, then a reduction otoplasty is in order. The oversized auricle presents an interesting dilemma. The circumference of the helical rim ultimately determines the shape and size of the auricular structure. When this situation presents itself, the area of both the helix and scapha must be reduced. This is readily

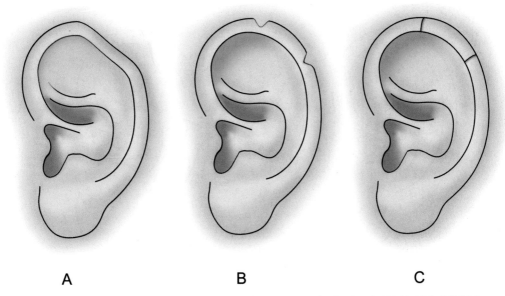

Figure 7-2. Treatment of a severely effaced helical rim. (A) Flattened helical curl. (B) Multiple full thickness helical wedge excisions, and (C) Primary closure to recreate a helical furl.

accomplished via removal of a segment of helical and scaphal cartilage and skin of up to 1 cm in length.

As with other cosmetic otoplasty techniques, helicoscaphal reductive methods were developed for reconstructive purposes for the treatment of microtia and chondrocutaneous malignancies of the ear. Tanzer[2] has reviewed various patterns of wedge and crescentic excisions (**Figure 7-3**). These have been further elaborated upon by various authors[3,4]. Although they were advanced for other purposes, these techniques are equally applicable to the reduction of the helical perimeter for cosmetic means. However, these maneuvers are to be avoided unless the deformity is significant, since troublesome scarring may result from helical and scaphal excisions. While these scars are potentially acceptable to reconstructive patients, those patients in search of purely cosmetic improvements are likely to be more discerning.

The methods described above are all really variations on a theme, each designed to decrease the concentric area of the helix and scapha via excision, while minimizing incident cartilaginous deformities. All provide for bipedicled chondrocutaneous helical advancement flaps for suitable closure of the resultant defect. Of these options, we prefer to use a modification of the inverted offset pentagonal wedge excision, if necessary (**Figure 7-4**). This allows for a

versatile excision of anterior skin and cartilage while reducing tension at the suture line. Construction of a model of the smaller ear with exposed radiograph allows us accurate determination of the amount of scaphal reduction desired, and it permits easy intraoperative comparison between ears.

Hinderer[5] has stressed the importance of placing the skin and cartilage incisions at different levels to avoid notching of the helical rim. Potential for this complication is greater when the skin suture line overlies the point of weakness at the location of the cartilaginous incision. This step at the junction of the helical rim and scapha breaks up the incision, and it is important for scar camouflage and prevention of scar contracture across the helical rim. In addition to offsetting these incisions, a stair-step approach to incision of the helical rim cartilage may be considered as an added measure of security. Also of importance is the need to cut back the cartilage slightly more than the skin, so that the skin suture line is not under tension. The planned skin excision should be just enough to eliminate redundancy.

The incision is made perpendicular to the long axis of the helix and carried through anterior skin and cartilage. The posterior skin is initially left intact. Since major blood supply to the auricle passes from posteriorly-based perforating arterial branches, there is no serious risk of vascular compromise with this approach. A corresponding offset wedge of

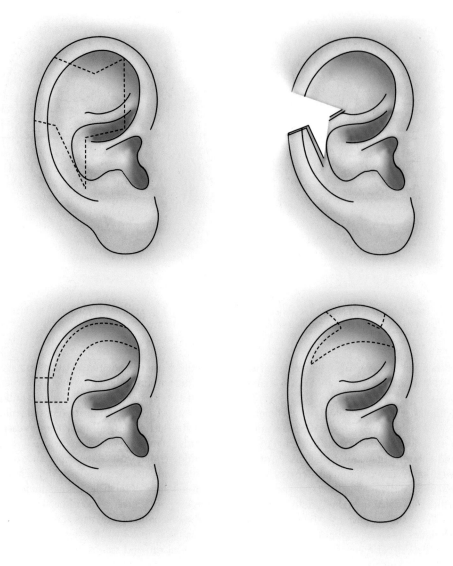

Figure 7-3. Various scaphal wedge and crescentic full thickness excisions for treatment of an enlarged scapha.

scaphal cartilage is then removed and surrounding skin is undermined to assist with re-drapage. The scaphal incisions are extended superiorly and inferiorly at the junction of the helical rim to facilitate helical bipedicled advancement flap closure. The cartilaginous arch is then reconstituted by suturing of the cut cartilage edges with 4-0 polyglactin (Vicryl), or polydioxanone (PDS) although some authors prefer permanent suture for this purpose. The rim is secured to the free edge of the scapha as well. Often, it is necessary to excise a Burow's triangle of redundant skin from the posterior (medial)

surface. Alternatively, for large reductions, the medial skin can be removed primarily at the same time as excision of the lateral skin and full thickness cartilage excision as a planned fusiform scaphal reduction.

Lobular Abnormalities

Medialization of a Protruding Lobule

Excessive protrusion of the ear lobe is a common feature of the prominent auricle. Failure to correct

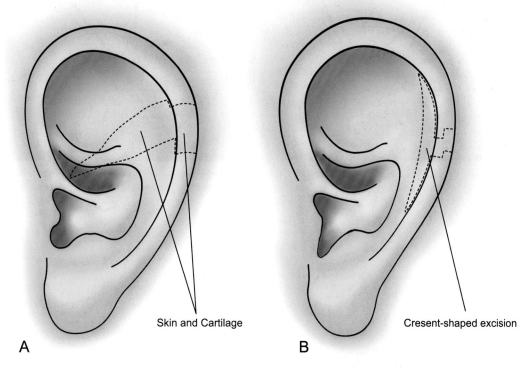

Skin and Cartilage

Cresent-shaped excision

A

B

Figure 7-4. Our preferred treatment of an enlarged scapha. (A) Modified offset pentagonal wedge excision with offset of helical and scaphal excisions to prevent notching of the helical rim (B) Alternatively, crescent-shaped scaphal excision with stair-step approach to helical excision.

lobular protrusion during otoplasty in the setting of a corrected cartilaginous framework will cause this deformity to appear even more conspicuous. As we touched on in the previous chapter, this problem may usually be attributed to one of several underlying anatomic features[6]. Most often, a prolonged or protrusive cauda helicis is anchoring and, in fact, dragging the lobule laterally. At other times, excess fibrofatty tissue of the lobule itself is responsible for causing the lobule to appear laterally protrusive.

As a consequence, a number of techniques need to be applied in order to resolve this distortion. Since the lobule is attached cranially to the helical framework, the problem may be controlled indirectly in a small subset of patients simply by correction of the antihelix to draw the lobule medially. This was successfully achieved in 28 of 159 patients in the experience of Beernink and colleagues[7].

If there is a subtle protrusion, tailoring of the skin excision to involve a portion of retrolobular skin may be sufficient to achieve a suitable correction. The postauricular skin excision can be extended over the posterior surface of the lobule via an "open book" approach with a swallow-tail shaped configuration. Some have even suggested carrying this excision into the retrolobular sulcus; however, this process may inadvertently over-medialize the lobule and blunt the retrolobular sulcus. More often than not, soft tissue excision alone will artificially flatten the retrolobular fold under excessive tension, predisposing to loss of correction and the induction of postoperative keloid formation in this area.

A more reliable approach to this problem is to address the contribution of the cauda helicis. Access to this structure is attained via the extended postauricular incision wherein both the cauda helicis and medial concha are exposed (**Figure 7-5**). A single horizontal permanent mattress suture is placed, drawing the cauda helicis to the concha. Occasionally, the cauda helicis may be weakened by scoring methods or incised along its scaphal attachment prior to suturing (**Figure 7-6**). We do not advise, as some authors do, excision of the cauda helicis. Rather than capitalizing on this structure's ability to anchor the lobule, excision of the lobule's cranial

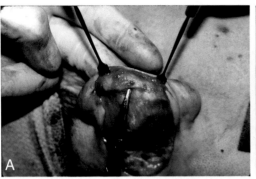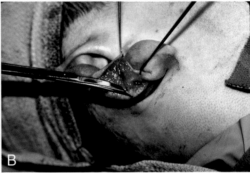

Figure 7-5. Intraoperative exposure of the cauda helicis via an extended postauricular incision. (A) Sharp separation of the cauda helix from its attachment to the concha; this may be sutured to the concha to medialize the lobule. (B) Incision of the cauda helix; we do not advise resection as this forfeits suture control of the lobule.

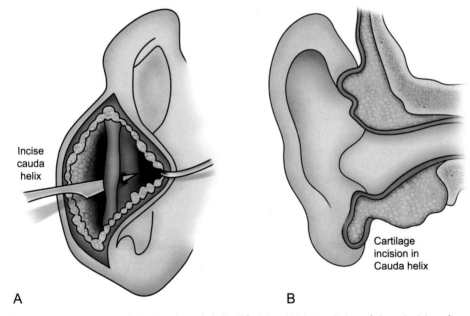

Figure 7-6. Diagramatic depiction of cauda helical incision. (A) Lateral view of sharp incision of the cauda helicis; this can be accomplished via the existing posterior incision. (B) Cross-sectional view showing the level of cauda helical incision.

attachment serves only to forfeit suture control of the lobule.

Siegert[6] further advocates a long-acting absorbable suture such as 5-0 polydioxanone (PDS) between the dermis of the lateral undersurface of the lobule and the cartilage of the cavum concha. A similar posteromedial suture placement is suggested by Spira[8]. Alternatively, the suture may be anchored to the mastoid periosteum as recommended by Gosain and Recinos[9]. Siegert advises use of multiple fixation points as necessary to modify the shape and position of the lobule, depending on the individual

malformation. By anchoring the sutures to the concha, a normal distance of about 18 to 20 mm can be established between the lobule and the skin overlying the mastoid process. If one utilizes this helpful maneuver, care must be taken to securely fix the suture in the lobular dermis to allow stabilization, but not so superficially so as to produce tethering or suture visibility. Additionally, the path of each arc of the mattress suture must be wide enough to permit strong anchorage of the intervening fibrofatty tissue of the lobule. In a slight modification, a small anterior stab incision may be made in the lobule to facilitate passage of the suture via an anterior or posterior approach. Siegert performs excision of only the redundant retrolobular skin after the lobule position has been achieved.

Reduction of an Enlarged Lobule

A large, dependent lobule is a recognized mark of the aging auricle and is a common feature of otoplasty among older women. This has been referred to as lobule-chalasis[6]. Most often, the unrelenting weight of the woman's preferred earring is the inciting cause. Sometimes, though, lobular elongation is seen as a result of poor positioning after rhytidectomy or parotidectomy. Finally, it may be seen congenitally even among younger women. Whatever the cause, an enlarged lobule is readily addressed contemporaneously with the otoplastic procedure.

Numerous techniques for reduction of an enlarged lobule have been described by authors such as Tanzer[2]. These primarily involve excision of a portion of the outer lobule with rotational flap mobilization of the remaining lobule for closure (**Figure 7-7**). This closure is facilitated by incorporation of a Burow's triangle excision as part of the initial planning. Siegert[6] advises an L-shaped excision of the inner lobule, adapted from Davis[10], preferring to conceal the incision along the attachment of the lobule to the cheek. This excision respects and preserves the lobular aesthetic subunit as a whole. To preserve lobular blood supply, the posterior skin is preserved intact. It does, however, create an attached lobule where none was before, so this must be aesthetically acceptable to the patient.

Danecke[2] described a novel approach for lobule reduction by doubling the lobe upon itself. The area of lobule to be reduced is marked on the posterior surface of the lobule and a partial thickness excision of posterior skin and subcutaneous fat is undertaken. The residual anterior skin and remnant fibrofatty tissue is then folded upon itself with the resultant scar hidden on the lobule's posterior surface. This is an interesting solution to the problem of a redundant lobule. However, it can be difficult to recreate a lobule with normal thickness and contour given the particular fibrous nature of the fibrofatty tissue in this area. Additionally, earring holes present a dilemma for this procedure, whereas the others presented allow for either direct excision or incorporation into the Burow's triangle.

We prefer a simple crescentic skin and soft tissue excision of the redundant portion of the lobule (**Figure 7-8**). Matching incisions are marked on both the anterior and posterior lobular surfaces to map out the desired curved shape for the new free edge of the lobule. A curved, dissecting tissue scissors is used to resect this tissue along a smooth, curvilinear plane. A strip of subcutaneous fat is further removed to facilitate closure of the skin edges. When the lobule is viewed from inferiorly, this excision should appear as a symmetric 'inverted V'. The incision is then easily closed without tension using a running 6-0 nylon closure. Sutures are retained in this location for 6 days to prevent scar widening or dehiscence. Clear advantages of this technique include the concealment of the scar on the posterior free edge of the lobule, and the ability to exactly and symmetrically gauge the degree of excision.

In this chapter, we have demonstrated the final refinements of our otoplasty technique, including treatment of helical, scaphal, and lobular abnormalities (**Figure 7-9**). In the next chapter, we will discuss nuances of wound closure, dressing care, and other aspects of postoperative management that are essential to provision of a satisfying otoplasty result.

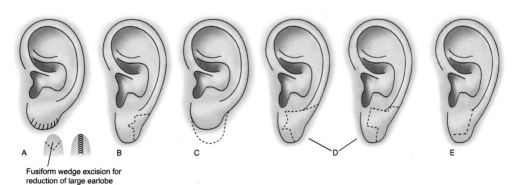

A

Fusiform wedge excision for
reduction of large earlobe

B   C   D   E

Figure 7-7. Various techniques for reduction of an enlarged lobule. (A) Burow's technique; (B) Joseph's technique; (C) Danecke's technique; (D) Tanzer's technique; (E) Davis' technique.

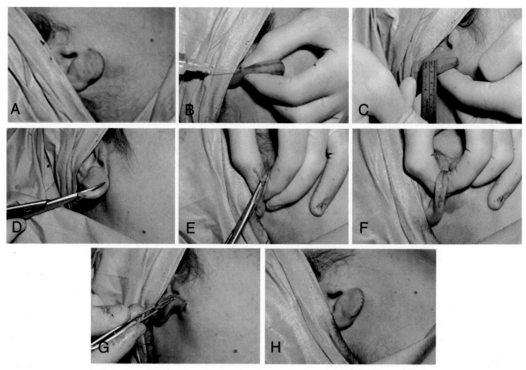

Figure 7-8. Intraoperative photos showing sequence of our preferred lobular reduction technique. (A) Marking of a crescentic full thickness lobular excision. (B) Infiltration of local anesthesia after marking. (C) Measuring to ensure symmetric anterior and posterior skin excision so that resultant scar falls along the lobular margin. (D) Sharp excision with a curved tissue scissors. (E) Further excision of a central rim of fat to allow for easy approximation of skin edges. (F) Tension-free approximation of skin, and (G) Simple running skin closure showing smooth lobular contour.

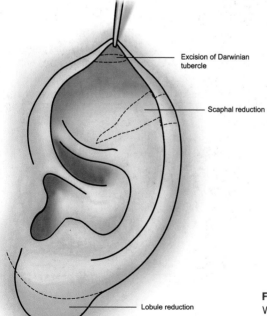

Excision of Darwinian tubercle

Scaphal reduction

Lobule reduction

Figure 7-9. Summary of otoplasty refinements. Wedge resections, lobule reduction, and helical trimming may be performed as desired.

References

1. Gibson T, Davis W. The distortion of autogenous cartilage grafts: its cause and prevention. *Br J Plast Surg* 10:257, 1958.
2. Tanzer RC. Deformities of the auricle: congenital deformities. In: Converse JM, ed. Reconstructive Plastic Surgery. Philadelphia: WB Saunders, pp. 1671–1719, 1977.
3. Songcharoen S, Smith RA, Jabaley ME. Tumors of the external ear and reconstruction of defects. *Clin Plast Surg* 5:447, 1978
4. Mellette JR jr. Ear reconstruction with local flaps. *J Dermatol Surg Oncol* 17:176, 1991.
5. Hinderer UT, del Rio JL, Fregenal FJ. Macrotia. *Aesthetic Plast Surg* 11:81, 1987.
6. Siegert R. Correction of the lobule. *Facial Plast Surg* 20(4):293–98, 2004.
7. Beernink JH, Blocksma R, Moore WD. The role of the helical tail in cosmetic otoplasty. *Plast Reconstr Surg* 64:115, 1979.
8. Spira M. Otoplasty: What I do now. A 30-year perspective. *Plast Reconstr Surg* 104(3):834–40, 1999.
9. Gosain AK, Recinos RF. A novel approach to correction of the prominent lobule during otoplasty. *Plast Reconstr Surg* 112(2):575–83, 2003.
10. Davis J. Aesthetic and reconstructive Otoplasty. New York: Springer, 150–59, 1987.

8

Closure, Dressings, and Postoperative Care

Peter A. Adamson, MD, FRCSC, FACS and
Jason A. Litner, MD, FRCSC

Introduction

We have discussed in a previous chapter various splinting materials and methods for nonsurgical attempts to remedy the prominent ear. These are notable in that they underscore the unique elastic nature of the auricular cartilage. These very properties work against the surgeon in promoting relapse and loss of correction beginning in the immediate postoperative period. For this reason and others, the postoperative ritual is especially significant in the eyes of otoplasty surgeons.

While skin closure and postoperative dressing of the surgical field is usually taken as an afterthought for most other plastic surgical procedures, it is not and should not be so when it comes to otoplasty. This is because careless or injudicious placement of dressings may predispose to disastrous results with this particular operation. These may include skin and cartilage necrosis owing to a too-tight dressing or to one that mistakenly folds over an edge of the auricle. An excessively constrictive dressing may also promote early infection and the dreaded chondritis. Asymmetry or distortion of the final outcome may result from uneven splinting of the newly formed auricles. Clumsy performance of skin closure may dispose the incision to dehiscence, suture extrusion, hypertrophic scarring, or keloid formation. Failure to attend to the patient in the early postoperative period may also cause one to miss a minor hematoma. Assiduous attention to detail and maintenance of focus is crucial in this phase of the operation, as it is in all others, to avoid such potential complications.

Surgical Technique

Closure and Dressing

Once the conchal and antihelical positions are established, we choose to close the postauricular incision with interrupted, inverted intracuticular 4-0 chromic gut sutures (**Figure 8-1**). We previously relied on 4-0 polyglactin (Vicryl) sutures for their longer period of tensional strength, but we have since abandoned this choice because of a greater incidence of delayed suture extrusion experienced with this material (**Figure 8-2**). The loose closure allows for egress of fluids, obviating the need for surgical drains. The wound is copiously irrigated with an antibiotic rinse prior to closure. The skin should readily drape into the postauricular sulcus

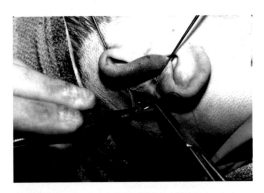

Figure 8-1. Skin closure with interrupted, buried, intracuticular 4-0 chromic gut sutures.

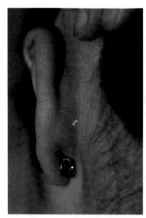

Figure 8-2. Vicryl suture extrusion.

without any attendant wound closing tension. The postauricular skin flap should be further undermined in the event that any tension is encountered or if the final location of the incision appears that it will overlie the Mustarde-type sutures. The knots of these Mustardé sutures should be pushed forward, as advised by Mustardé[1] himself, so they do not encroach on the incision line as this may engender suture complications.

Some authors would advise taking further precautions with incision planning and closure to minimize the risk of suture complications, inclusive of a 'bowstring' effect, skin thinning and ulceration, suture exposure, and suture extrusion. In a study comparing various otoplasty techniques and outcomes over a 5-year period, Mandal and colleagues[2] found a significantly diminished rate of suture complications when a posterior fascial flap was designed with a cartilage suturing technique as compared to a suturing or scoring technique without this added soft tissue coverage. While we find these results compelling, we have not yet found it necessary to incorporate this recommendation into our routine, since we have encountered these complications relatively infrequently.

Following completion of additional procedures as needed, we use bolsters of cotton soaked in equal parts hydrogen peroxide and mineral oil that are carefully molded to the folds of the auricle following application of antibiotic ointment (**Figure 8-3**). Plentiful soft fluff dressing is employed followed by application of a heavy compressive mastoid dressing with Kerlix cling wrap (**Figure 8-4**). The dressing is taped to the cheek area to prevent excessive movement and slippage. Extreme care is taken to avoid any pressure points that might predispose to skin necrosis.

In the case of our cartilage-sparing technique, the dressing serves several purposes. It conceals the wounds, maintains cleanliness, provides protection from minor external trauma, and imparts some splinting action for the new auricular contour. It cannot prevent a major hematoma, but it may mitigate minor blood and fluid collections and excessive soft tissue swelling, especially in the area of the posterior sulcus and the complex interstices of the lateral auricular surface. Stucker and colleagues[3] have noted that this wet-to-dry dressing type is of particular benefit in that the moisture is wicked away into the fluffed gauze as the cotton dries, creating a cast of the ear. For this reason, the dressing

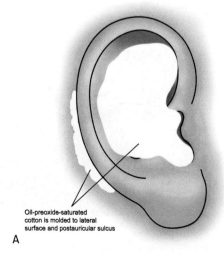

Oil-preoxide-saturated cotton is molded to lateral surface and postauricular sulcus

A

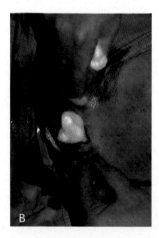

B

Figure 8-3. Oil-peroxide soaked cotton bolster. (A) Diagrammatic representation (B) Intraoperative photo.

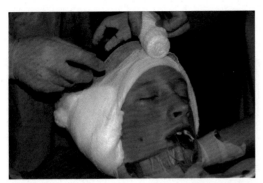

Figure 8-4. Placement of a bulky mastoid-type kerlix dressing.

is moistened prior to removal to decrease patient discomfort and potential injury.

For techniques that rely more heavily on isolated cartilage-incisional procedures, the conforming nature of the dressing plays an active participatory role in molding the final form of the ear. Nolst Trenité has advised that if, after final closure, the "contour of the new antihelix is not completely satisfying, additional external mattress sutures can be applied over adaptic rolls"[4]. He advises maintaining this dressing for a week as, no doubt, it possesses a very real function in helping to shape and maintain auricular position. In our graduated approach, this role is borne to a greater degree by the internal suture plication of the cartilage, rendering the duration of postoperative dressing of slightly lesser consequence, though certainly not trivial.

A wide variety of approaches to postoperative care exists for this procedure, some quite intricate. Aygit[5], for example, uses a custom-made mold for 2 weeks postoperatively. Azuara[6] similarly recommends a moldable porous polyester splint for 72 hours with a compressive dressing applied continuously for 1 week and nightly for 1 month. Bulstrode and colleagues[7] advise packing the folds of the auricle with cotton wool followed by application of elastic tape for 1 week for use with a percutaneous scoring otoplasty technique. The bulk of authors use a standard mastoid conforming dressing postoperatively for a variable period. To date, no investigations have correlated a difference in surgical outcomes with the choice of style or duration of the postoperative dressing.

Postoperative Care

Many authors do not disturb the dressing for 5 days or more postoperatively, removing it only for excessive complaints of pain or bleeding. In contrast,

we insist on removing the dressing on the first postoperative day to inspect the wounds. This facilitates early identification of complications such as skin ischemia or early hematoma formation. We believe this to be important since the best possible outcomes are more attainable with early intervention.

A somewhat lighter dressing is replaced and is worn for a further 4 days in children. This second dressing may be omitted for adults and cooperative older children. Following removal of the dressings, patients are instructed to wear an elastic athletic headband round the clock for 2 weeks postoperatively, and then nightly for 2 weeks more. This is especially important in the prevention of accidental nocturnal injury that might disrupt the sutures. There is no need for removal of the absorbable sutures. For 6 weeks, patients are discouraged from any rough play or circumstances that might otherwise lead to traumatic distraction of the auricle, since a history of external trauma has been associated with about half of the cases of recurrence requiring revisional surgery[8].

Patients are given general education regarding cleansing and application of bactericidal ointment to the incisions, which may begin after dressing removal. Patients are instructed to avoid manipulation of the ears or any other activity that might predispose to a complicated course of healing. Light activities may resume almost immediately and aerobic exercise may recommence after 2 to 3 weeks. The complex interlocking stresses of the auricular cartilage that were broken down at surgery take some time to regain their strength and stability, although a precise timeline for adequate remodeling to occur is unknown. Presumably, a 6 to 8 week window provides sufficient time for remodeling and for soft tissue scarring to provide some external stability. This is why most surgeons will allow for stoppage of external pressure devices and for more vigorous activities to resume after this time, although every care should be taken indefinitely where the potential for direct trauma is concerned. No other restrictions are placed on the patient.

This chapter concludes our detailed description of our preferred graduated approach to otoplasty. Representative examples of this technique applied in adults and children are shown in **Figures 8-5 to 8-18**. In the next section, we will discuss controversies related to otoplasty techniques, and we will outline a diversity of practices from prominent international otoplasty surgeons, many quite different from our own. Although we cannot possibly hope to cover the whole multiplicity of available methods (after all, there are almost 200 known variations and counting), we will highlight the findings from large series of patients that run the gamut of available cartilage scoring, cutting, and combination techniques.

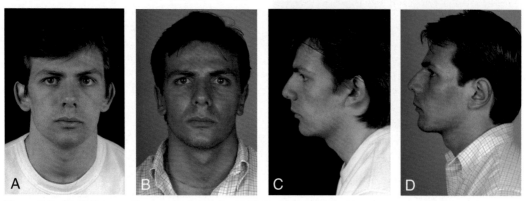

Figure 8-5. (A,C) Preoperative lop ear deformity (B,D) Postoperative results using our graduated cartilage-sparing otoplasty technique.

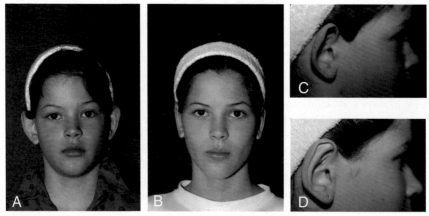

Figure 8-6. (A,C) Preoperative lop ear deformity (B,D) Postoperative results using our graduated cartilage-sparing otoplasty technique.

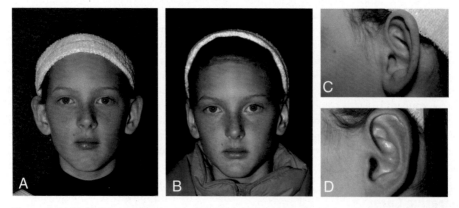

Figure 8-7. (A,C) Preoperative lop ear deformity (B,D) Postoperative results using our graduated cartilage-sparing otoplasty technique.

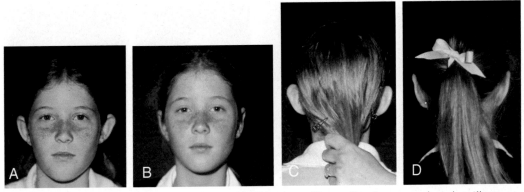

Figure 8-8. (A,C) Preoperative lop ear deformity (B,D) Postoperative results using our graduated cartilage-sparing otoplasty technique.

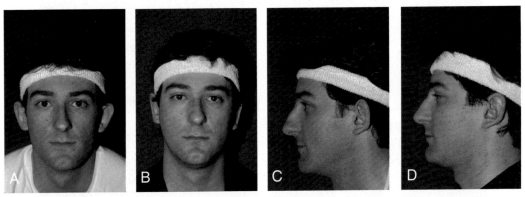

Figure 8-9. (A,C) Preoperative lop ear deformity (B,D) Postoperative results using our graduated cartilage-sparing otoplasty technique.

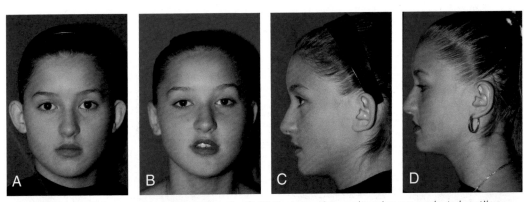

Figure 8-10. (A,C) Preoperative lop ear deformity (B,D) Postoperative results using our graduated cartilage-sparing otoplasty technique.

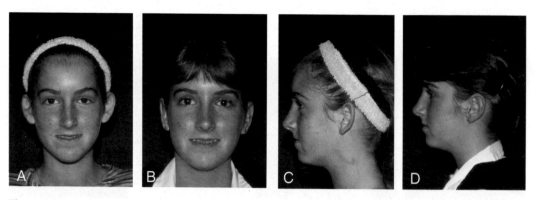

Figure 8-11. (A,C) Preoperative lop ear deformity (B,D) Postoperative results using our graduated cartilage-sparing otoplasty technique.

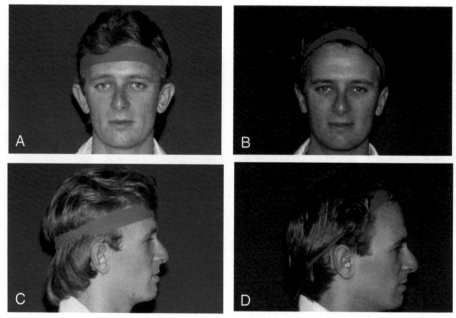

Figure 8-12. (A,C) Preoperative lop ear deformity (B,D) Postoperative results using our graduated cartilage-sparing otoplasty technique.

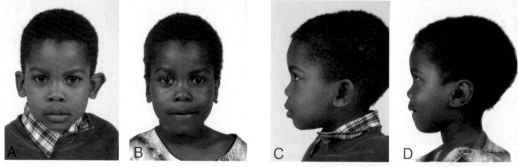

Figure 8-13. (A,C) Preoperative lop ear deformity (B,D) Postoperative results using our graduated cartilage-sparing otoplasty technique.

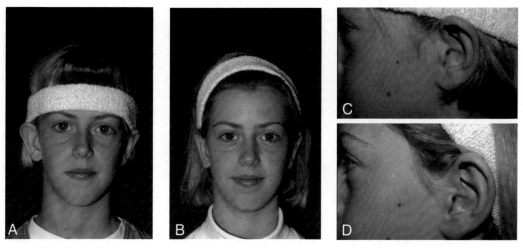

Figure 8-14. (A,C) Preoperative lop ear deformity (B,D) Postoperative results using our graduated cartilage-sparing otoplasty technique.

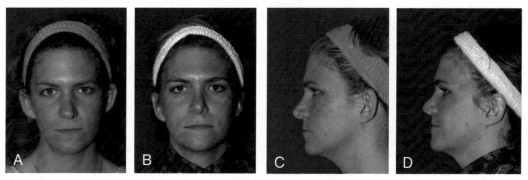

Figure 8-15. (A,C) Preoperative lop ear deformity (B,D) Postoperative results using our graduated cartilage-sparing otoplasty technique.

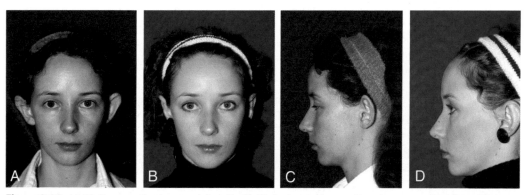

Figure 8-16. (A,C) Preoperative lop ear deformity (B,D) Postoperative results using our graduated cartilage-sparing otoplasty technique.

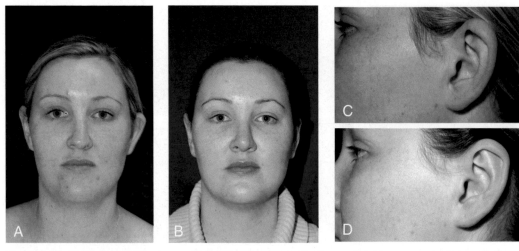

Figure 8-17. (A,C) Preoperative lop ear deformity (B,D) Postoperative results using our graduated cartilage-sparing otoplasty technique.

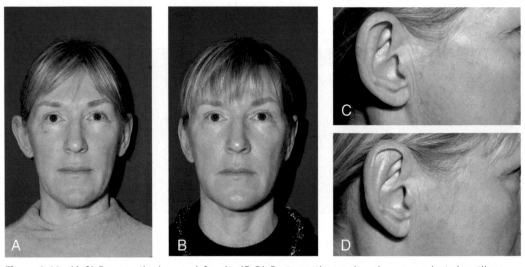

Figure 8-18. (A,C) Preoperative lop ear deformity (B,D) Postoperative results using our graduated cartilage-sparing otoplasty technique.

References

1. Mustarde JC. The correction of prominent ears using simple mattress sutures. *Br J Plast Surg;* 16:170, 1963.
2. Mandal A, Bahia H, Ahmad T, Stewart KJ. Comparison of cartilage scoring and cartilage sparing otoplasty: a study of 203 cases. *Plast Reconstr Aesthet Surg* 59(11):1170–6, 2006.
3. Burningham AR, Stucker FJ. Otoplasty technique: how I do it. *Facial Plast Surg Clin N Am* 14:73–77, 2006.
4. Nolst Trenité GJ. Otoplasty: a modified anterior scoring technique. *Facial Plast Surg* 20(4):277–85, 2004.
5. Aygit AC. Molding the ears after anterior scoring and concha repositioning: a combined approach for protruding ear correction. *Aesthetic Plast Surg* 27(1): 77–81, 2003.
6. Azuara E. Aesthetic otoplasty with remodeling of the antihelix for the correction of the prominent ear: criteria and personal technique. *Arch Facial Plast Surg;* 2(1):57–61, 2000.
7. Bulstrode NW, Huang S, Martin DL. Otoplasty by percutaneous anterior scoring. Another twist to the story: a long-term study of 114 patients. *Br J Plast Surg* 56(2):145–9, 2003.
8. Adamson PA, McGraw BL, Tropper GJ. Otoplasty: critical review of clinical results. *Laryngoscope* 101(8): 883–88, 1991.

9

SELECTED CARTILAGE-CUTTING OTOPLASTY TECHNIQUES

PETER A. ADAMSON, MD, FRCSC, FACS AND
JASON A. LITNER, MD, FRCSC

Introduction

Since the original descriptions of cartilage-splitting otoplasty techniques, culminating with the mid-century popularization of the Converse otoplasty, preference for a cutting-only technique has waned among the current generation of facial plastic surgeons. The tendency for such methods to produce unsightly cartilage ridging may explain this trend. However, more aggressive cutting techniques have not fallen completely by the wayside because of the correct assertion by their proponents that cartilage-sparing techniques, used alone, may favor a higher rate of recurrence of the original deformity. Cartilage-cutting techniques, to draw a distinction, may ensure a more lasting correction because the cartilage spring is permanently broken (**Figure 9-1**).

In the post-Mustardé era, most authors have supported a blending of techniques to form a hybrid approach. So, now, a cartilage-cutting label is assigned to any approach that routinely incorporates a full-thickness transcartilaginous incision or excision for the recreation of a correct antihelical or conchal contour. While destabilization of the cartilaginous framework may be sufficient for the purist, many surgeons choose to marry cutting maneuvers with post-transection suture stabilization.

Most modern cartilage-splitting techniques are derivatives of the advances put forth by Converse[1], Chongchet[2], and Crikelair[3]; that is to say, they involve some form of cartilaginous incision within the scapha, followed by tubing of the cartilage to form an antihelix with or without scoring to weaken its consistency. Select modern renditions of these techniques are outlined below.

Surgical Technique

The Method of Siegert

Siegert's preferred otoplasty procedure[4] is, at its core, a modification of the Converse technique. It entails a retroauricular approach with complete mobilization of the posterior surface of the auricular cartilage via a postauricular incision performed 1 cm medial to the helical margin. The lines of the intended cartilaginous incisions are marked with needles by pinning the cartilage through the anterior skin. A total of three incisions are made through posterior perichondrium and cartilage, along the posterior border of the antihelix, the anterior border of the superior crus, and the fold of the conchal rim (**Figure 9-2**). The anterior perichondrium is

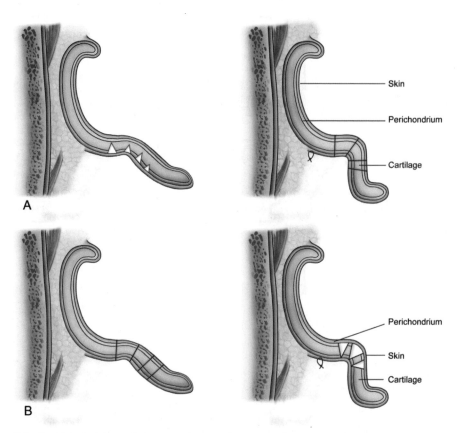

Figure 9-1. Cartilage incision techniques to alter cartilage spring. (A) Posterior incisions (B) Anterior incisions.

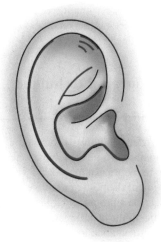

Figure 9-2. The method of Siegert. Projection onto the anterior auricle of the three posterior incomplete cartilage incisions. Weakening of the posterior perichondrium of the superior crus is undertaken to facilitate folding. Tubing of the cartilage is fixed with permanent suture.

preserved in its entirety. The posterior perichondrium may be weakened by scoring at the superior crus to facilitate folding.

Tubing of the antihelical cartilage is accomplished by pressure placed on the scapha. The curvature is fixed by placement of 4-0 Mersilene permanent sutures just above and just below the intercrural bifurcation to set the superior antihelix, with additional sutures placed as necessary to fix the inferior antihelix.

Conchal excess is treated by cartilage excision medial to the previously made conchal rim incision. If conchal prominence persists, it may be necessary to perform what Siegert calls a cavum rotation, or what is essentially conchal medialization in the manner of Furnas[5]. Retroauricular soft tissue is excised in order to allow this rotation to take place. Two or three resorbable 4-0 Vicryl sutures achieve fixation of the concha. Occasionally, the posterior auricular spine or other protrusive structures must be shaved with a scalpel. Conservative skin excision is deferred until the conclusion of the case. Finally, a specialized foam rubber dressing is applied for 7 days.

Siegert favors this cartilage-splitting technique because he feels that the excessive time required for cartilage fibers to remodel permits only the softest of auricular frameworks to be trusted to pure suture techniques. For this reason, permanent sutures are preferred to bind the antihelix. More reliable shaping can be assured by scoring of the most tension-bearing regions of the cartilage after bending, at least on the posterior surface. Only when the cartilage is overly sturdy does Siegert take the added step of transecting the cartilage to mobilize and score the anterior surface. In this setting, numerous superficial scores help to define the antihelix, which is, more or less, Crikelair's technique. In contrast to the stabilization of the antihelix, absorbable sutures are adequate for the conchamastoid sutures since the soft tissue scar necessary for stabilization in this area occurs far more rapidly than the cartilage remodeling required of the antihelix.

In a series of 210 patients treated over a 5-year period, Siegert and colleagues[4] reported stable and satisfying results utilizing this reliable and reproducible technique.

The Method of Nachlas

Nachlas[6] originally described his preferred otoplasty technique in 1970, which is loosely based on the prior work of Cloutier[7]. The arc of the intended neo-antihelix is tattooed on the skin with methylene blue-stained needles. A postauricular incision is then undertaken along this arc, with excision of an elliptical or hourglass-shaped slice of skin. Wide undermining of the postauricular skin is performed, followed by an incision through the auricular cartilage with a Cottle knife. The incision is located about 5 mm anterior to the tattoo marks indicating the apex of the new antihelix. Nachlas recommends resection of the cauda helicis to prevent postoperative bowing of the lobule. Next, triangular wedges are excised at the superior and inferior ends of the cartilage incision to facilitate rolling (**Figure 9-3**).

The anterior perichondrium is elevated off the surface of the cartilage for a distance of about 1 cm. The medial edge of the cartilage is then burred with a diamond abrader over the antihelix and the superior crus. The anterior surface of the lateral cartilage is also beveled and the medial edge is positioned overlying the lateral edge.

This is a true cartilage-splitting technique in that the cartilage edges are not secured with suture. Instead, the technique relies exclusively on the contouring procedure to maintain the auricle's altered position. The skin is closed simply using a running subcuticular suture. Nachlas minimizes the possibility of visible surface irregularities with this technique because of the position of the overlapping segments. In this manner, the free cartilage edge is facing posteriorly while the surface detectable on anterior view is the smooth convexity created by the new antihelix. Weakening of the cartilage superstructure via this combination of maneuvers greatly lowers the risk of reprotrusion.

The Method of Walter

The foundation of cartilage-splitting techniques is the notion that strategic division of the cartilage helps to curtail the intrinsic tension within the framework. Early work by Sercer[8], in 1951, and by Pollet[9], in 1957, centered on the idea of separating the helical segment from the antihelical segment of the auricle as a means to reduce this intrinsic tension. Walter[10] first published his incision-excision technique in 1958 in German, and in the English language literature in 1969. This method focused on division of these segments followed by remodeling of the antihelical, helical, and lobular fragments. The auricular cartilage is divided into three main segments: the helical section, including the cauda helicis; the antihelical section, including the superior and inferior crus; and, the concha. The originally described technique has been further adapted by Heppt[11].

In order to separate the pinna into component parts, the procedure consists of multiple incisions and excisions (**Figure 9-4**). The operation commences with a conventional postauricular incision and undermining to within 1 cm of the mastoid to avoid obliteration of the postauricular sulcus. Here is where convention stops. A transcartilaginous incision is made along the helical rim and along the medial aspect of the intended antihelix. These incisions are joined superiorly and inferiorly in a rounded fashion, resulting in complete separation of the auricular framework with a floating central segment and separation of the helical tail from the remaining structure. Further weakening of the cartilaginous spring is accomplished by wide undermining of the anterior aspect of the helical rim and amputation of the anterior helical ligament at the root of the helix.

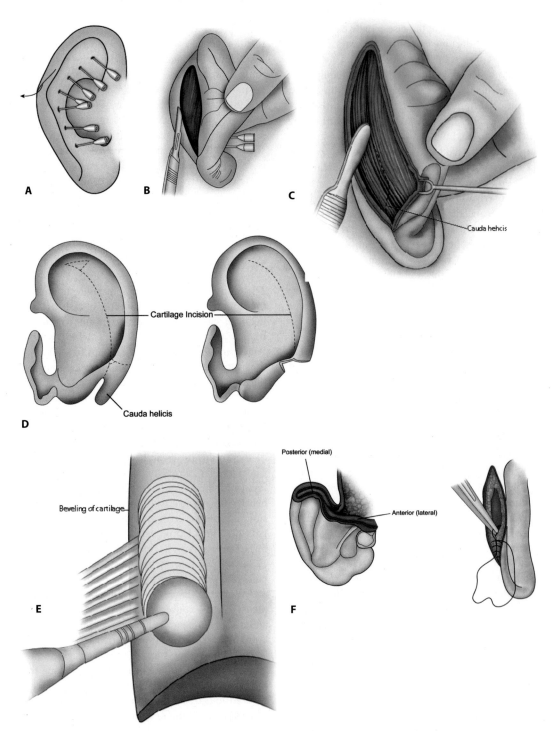

Figure 9-3. The method of Nachlas. (A) Line of the intended antihelix is tattooed with methylene blue using transcutaneous needle placement. (B) Postauricular skin excision is performed. (C) Cartilage is incised posteriorly after wide undermining approximately 4 mm lateral to the tattoo marks. (D) Inverted triangular cartilage excisions at each end of the cartilage incision with resection of the cauda helicis to facilitate cartilage overlap. (E) Beveling of the anterior aspect of the lateral and medial cartilaginous flap with a diamond burr until furling occurs, and (F) overlapping of the lateral and medial cartilage segments followed by skin closure.

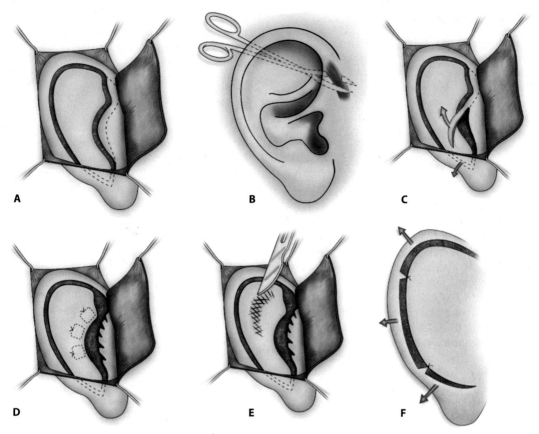

Figure 9-4. The method of Walter with adaptation by Heppt. (A) Retroauricular cartilage incision along entire helical rim and medial antihelical fold. (B) Transection of the anterior helical ligament. (C) Excision of conchal and helical cartilage to correct a prominent concha or lobule. (D) Vertical cuts in the concha to prevent ridging with optional antihelical mattress sutures. (E) Cross-hatched thinning of the posterior cartilage to accentuate the antihelix, and (F) Excision of redundant postauricular skin.

It is possible to injure the superficial temporal artery and vein by dissection in this area.

If there is a high conchal wall or prominent lobule, a strip of helical and conchal cartilage is excised. Small vertical cuts are created at the free edge of the conchal cartilage to mitigate the potential for a sharp edge in this area. In a departure from Walter's description, Heppt suggests that the new antihelix may be reinforced by placement of three mattress sutures to create a narrower fold, although this is generally reserved for situations in which there is an overly broad or sharply ridged antihelix produced by the above incisions. Final refinements may include thinning of the posterior aspect of the superior crus with cross-hatched incisions to generate greater definition. A persistently prominent lobule may be treated by incision or excision of the helical tail, trimming of the antitragus, or dovetailing the skin excision on the posterior surface of the lobule. Careful excision of the retroauricular skin comprises the final step in this operation.

This procedure represents a classic cartilage-cutting technique, wherein the break in the cartilage spring makes possible posterior rotation and furling of the auricular cartilage, without tension and without the need for further adjusting sutures. The main advantage of this method is that it may be applied to yield-pleasing aesthetic results in even the most difficult cases of stiff and unyielding cartilage or in revisional cases. Because the postauricular soft tissue is not dissected and conchal setback is not performed, the postauricular sulcus is completely preserved. As with all complex cartilage-splitting maneuvers, however, these should be reserved for experienced otoplastic surgeons to avoid the creation of visible irregularities by incorrect placement of incisions.

The Method of Pitanguy

Pitanguy[12] first reported his innovative 'island flap' technique for correction of 'fan-like' ears in 1961, and again in the English language literature a year later[13]. In this technique, the desired antihelical fold is marked at its apex by use of gentian violet through-and-through the skin and cartilage. On the posterior aspect of the pinna, a 1 cm dermal 'spindle' is removed and the posterior skin is undermined to the helical rim. A cartilage island is dissected free, consisting of a segment roughly 2 mm wide surrounding the previously marked arc and simulating the preferred antihelical line. This island is luxated ventrally (anteriorly) and fixed temporarily in this position with a needle cannula placed through the curvature of the antihelix. This fixation is rendered permanent by placement of 3-0 absorbable sutures connecting the cut medial and lateral cartilaginous cut edges. Conchal redundancy is treated by conchal rotation via placement of a concha-mastoid suture, affixing it to the mastoid periosteum. Finally, the skin is closed and dressings are applied.

In comparison to the cartilage-cutting procedures summarized above, the Pitanguy 'island flap' technique is a relatively simple procedure that is reliably replicated. For that reason, it has been often imitated and modified by numerous authors. Pitanguy himself reported on a 25-year experience[14] with this technique in 488 cases, demonstrating a lasting aesthetic correction with preservation of an attractive scaphaconchal angle and having few short-term or long-term complications.

Werdin and colleagues[15] recently reported on their adaptation of this technique in 278 patients over a 15-year period. Modifications included conchal resection as opposed to posterior suture rotation of the concha, and added support of the antihelical fold by mattress sutures in the case of rigid ears. Complications were recorded in 7% of patients with 4% requiring operative revision. The most frequent complications were relapse (3%), telephone ear (1%), and reverse telephone ear (<1%).

The low recurrence rate associated with this technique is attributed to the configuration of the related cartilage segments that are created. The cartilage island technique itself consistently interrupts the intrinsic cartilage tension. Residual strength is partly overcome by the mattress sutures. In contrast to Converse's technique, the wide area of scar generated between the ventral cartilaginous island and the coapted dorsal cartilage serves to further reinforce the correction. If not applied with extreme care, this technique can result in postoperative deformations of the pinna and associated asymmetry. However, in experienced hands, it has produced quite favorable outcomes and enthusiasm for the 'island flap' technique is shared by others[16,17].

The Method of Bauer

While most otoplasty techniques center on treatment of the underdeveloped antihelix, Bauer and colleagues[18] concentrate their attention on correction of conchal hypertrophy via chondrocutaneous resection. They have made the concha their focus because they have noted the majority of patients presenting for secondary otoplasty to be those whose conchal hypertrophy had been missed or undertreated, often resulting in a so-called 'hidden helix' deformity when the antihelix is treated aggressively. Thus, for these authors, the concha is the key anatomic feature to be addressed in the prominent ear with or without a traditional posterior approach to the antihelix (**Figure 9-5**).

In this procedure, an incision is made anteriorly within the concha at the junction of the horizontal floor and vertical wall, and is carried through anterior skin and conchal cartilage. It is the authors' belief that too high placement of the incision can lead to unsightly scarring and to loss of control of the anterior antihelical border, potentially complicating creation of a smooth antihelical relief. The amount of conchal excess can be estimated by gentle pressure with setback of the antihelix. A crescentic segment of anterior skin and cartilage is excised. More cartilage than skin is removed to ensure a tension-free closure. After the desired excision is complete, the cartilaginous edges are reapproximated with interrupted 5-0 clear nylon sutures and the skin incision is closed in two layers.

The antihelix and lobule are then addressed as needed via a retroauricular "squid"-shaped skin excision. This is a modification of the traditional dumbbell-shaped excision with the inferior end widened into a diamond shape to address the prominent lobule. The maximal width of the lower extent of this excision is positioned at the point of maximal lobule prominence. This superior excision is designed to allow suture placement to correct both upper and lower pole prominence. The posterior conchal bowl and scapha is exposed via supraperichondrial undermining. The perichondrium is preserved in an effort to reduce the chances for suture pull-through. Separation of the cartilaginous helical tail from the helical rim during this

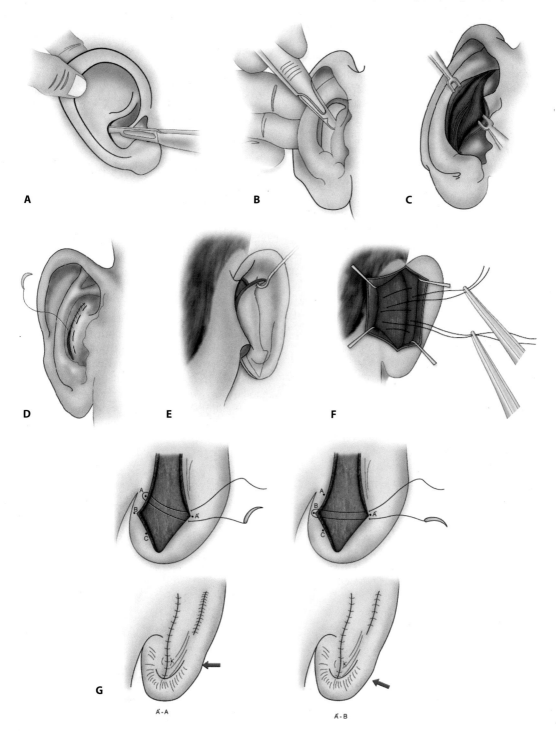

Figure 9-5. The method of Bauer. (A) Conchal skin incision located at the interface of the conchal floor and vertical wall. (B) Crescent-shaped chondrocutaneous segment removed with more cartilage than skin excised. (C) Cartilage edges approximated with 5-0 clear nylon. (D) Skin closed in two layers. (E) Squid-shaped posterior skin excision to allow suture placement for correction of upper, mid, and lower ear prominence. (F) Placement of scaphamastoid fascia sutures. (G) Skin incision closed and appropriate lobular contour determined by varying initial suture position with A′ sutured to either A, B, or C followed by running closure.

dissection will facilitate later correction of lobular prominence.

Bauer and colleagues recommend subsequent placement of scaphal-mastoid and helical sulcus-mastoid 4-0 clear nylon sutures to recreate a helical fold once it has been temporarily set back with Keith needles. Finally, the skin defect is closed primarily with 5-0 chromic gut sutures. The appropriate contour and projection of the lobule are set by strategic initial suture placement to create the desired shape. The remaining skin closure is performed in a running fashion.

Bauer and colleagues[18] reported on their results with this technique in 47 patients operated on over a 7-year period, with follow-up ranging from 6 months to 7 years. Three complications required revision, all of which constituted early relapses at the upper pole, which were corrected with replacement scaphamastoid sutures. A survey of both patients and parents at the 1-year postoperative mark revealed universal postoperative satisfaction. The anterior conchal incision reportedly healed well and was concealed by shadows cast within the conchal bowl. There was no incidence of keloid formation in this series. The sometimes bothersome skin folding that occurs within the conchal bowl after isolated conchal cartilage excision is prevented in this technique by the inclusion of anterior skin excision[19]. The potential for recurrent conchal hypertrophy is practically eliminated in contradistinction to the possibility for recurrent conchal prominence when conchamastoid sutures are disrupted.

Other Notable Cutting Techniques

An alternative to conchal setback for treatment of the abnormally angulated concha is the conchal flap advocated by Spira[20]. In this technique, the medial concha is incised and a laterally based conchal cartilage flap is developed and sutured to the mastoid process (**Figure 9-6**). This maneuver reliably reduces the conchamastoid angle with a negligible residual conchal bowl defect. In the authors' hands, this method is usually applied in conjunction with a typical suture technique for treatment of the antihelix. A somewhat different conchal flap technique is advocated by Elliot[21] in order to treat a hypertrophic conchal bowl (**Figure 9-7**).

Park[22] has taken this idea one step further by advocating posterior 'tumbling' of a similar conchal cartilage flap underneath the posterior auricular skin and affixing it to the posterior lidded helix or scapha for correction of the lop ear deformity.

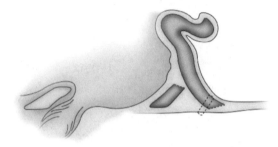

Figure 9-6. Lateral conchal flap setback technique. The laterally based conchal flap is sutured to the mastoid fascia to allow setback without compromising the auditory canal.

An anterior or posterior approach may be used for this purpose. The elastic recoil created by the flap's conchal side forcibly pulls the lidded helix into an erect position, increasing the vertical height of the auricle. Moderate lop ear deformity may be satisfactorily treated in this manner.

Jammet and colleagues[23] reported in the French literature on results of a cartilage-splitting technique that they term a partial anterior chondrotomy. In their estimation, 95% of results were considered good or very good. The advantages of partial anterior chondrotomy are also supported by others[24].

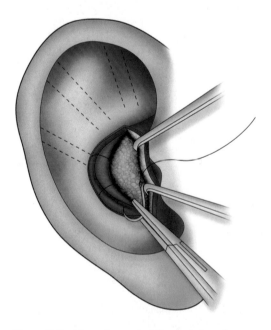

Figure 9-7. Alternate conchal flap technique for correction of conchal hypertrophy. The medial conchal cartilage is incised, overlapped laterally, and sutured. The auditory meatus is preserved.

Balogh and Millesi[26] studied 77 patients who had undergone otoplasty via a cartilage excision method 15 to 25 years earlier to determine whether any auricular growth alterations had occurred. The mean age at time of surgery was 7.2 years. Standard morphometric variables were compared with 200 control ears. There was no statistical difference in auriculocephalic angle, indicating that the desired setback had been maintained. Morphologic parameters were not significantly divergent on most measures with the surgical group having a significantly larger ear width and significantly smaller ear length. Operated ears were larger than control ears in all other dimensions. The authors concluded that auricular growth was not impaired by cartilage-cutting otoplasty performed in childhood.

Cartilage-cutting methods have been much criticized for the associated threat of major postoperative distortions. As noted in this chapter, however, application of classical cartilage-cutting techniques can lead to dependably positive outcomes in experienced hands. In the next chapter, we will review the host of otoplasty techniques that rely chiefly on scoring maneuvers to achieve a natural auricular contour.

References

1. Converse JM, Nigro A, Wilson FA, Johnson N. A technique for surgical correction of lop ears. *Plast Reconstr Surg* 15:411, 1955.
2. Chongchet V. A method for antihelix reconstruction. *Br J Plast Surg* 16:268, 1963.
3. Ju DM, Li C, Crikelair GF. The surgical correction of protruding ears. *Plast Reconstr Surg* 32:283, 1963.
4. Mattheis S, Siegert R. The modified Converse technique in combination with cavum rotation. *Facial Plast Surg* 20(4):271–5, 2004.
5. Furnas DW. Correction of prominent ears by conchamastoid sutures. *Plast Reconstr Surg* 42:189, 1968.
6. Nachlas NE, Duncan D, Trail M. Otoplasty. *Arch Otolaryngol* 91:44, 1970.
7. Cloutier AM. Correction of outstanding ears. *Plast Reconstr Surg* 28:412, 1961.
8. Sercer A. Notes on the cause and correlation of protruding ears. *Pract Otorhinolaryngol Basel* 13:9–16, 1951.
9. Pollet J. Plicature de l'antihélix pour la correction des oreilles mal formées. *Ann Chir Plast* 2:207–12, 1957.
10. Walter C. Plastic correction of lop ears. *Z Laryngol Rhinol Otol* 37(1):27–33,1958.
11. Walter C. Reconstructive procedures on the auricle. *Trans Am Acad Ophthalmol Otolaryngol* 73(2):266–73,1969.
12. Heppt WJ. The Incision-Excision technique in minor auricular deformities. *Facial Plast Surg* 20(4):287–92, 2004.
13. Pitanguy I, Rebelo C. Fan-like ears: considerations on the problem and suggestion of a personal technic. *Rev Bras Cir* 42:267–77, 1961.
14. Pitanguy I, Rebello C. Ansiform ears: correction by "island" technique. *Acta Chir Plast* 4:267–77, 1962.
15. Pitanguy I, Müller P, Piccolo N, Ramalho E, Solinas R. The treatment of prominent ears: a 25-year survey of the island technique. *Aesthetic Plast Surg* 11(2):87–93, 1987.
16. Werdin F, Wolters M, Lampe H. Pitanguy's otoplasty: report of 551 operations. *Scand J Plast Reconstr Surg Hand Surg* 41:283–7, 2007.
17. DeMoura LF. Correcting prominent ears with the island technique. *Trans Sect Otolaryngol Am Acad Ophthalmol Otolaryngol* 84(5):898–903, 1977.
18. Bartkowski SB, Szuta M, Zapala J. Pitanguy's method of protruding ear correction from our own experience: review of 80 cases. *Aesthetic Plast Surg* 25(2):103–10, 2001.
19. Bauer BS, Song DH, Aitken ME. Combined otoplasty technique: chondrocutaneous conchal resection as the cornerstone to correction of the prominent ear. *Plast Reconstr Surg* 110(4):1033–40, 2002.
20. Smith R, Dickinson JT, Teachey WS. Medial conchal excision in otoplasty. *Laryngoscope* 85(4):738–50, 1975.
21. Spira M, Stal S. The conchal flap: an adjunct in otoplasty. *Ann Plast Surg* 11(4):291–8, 1983.
22. Elliott RA Jr. Complications in the treatment of prominent ears. *Clin Plast Surg* 5(3):479–90, 1978.
23. Park C. The tumbling concha-cartilage flap for correction of the lop ear. *Plast Reconstr Surg* 106(2): 259–65, 2000.
24. Jammet P, Atlan G, Cisotto J, Souyris F. Partial anterior chondrotomy in the correction of prominent ears: apropos of 140 re-examined cases. *Ann Chir Plast Esthet* 37(2):182–8, 1992.
25. Labbé D, Siama M, Rigot-Jolivet M, Compère JF. Partial anterior chondrotomy for correction of protruding ears. *Rev Stomatol Chir Maxillofac* 87(6):389–93, 1986.
26. Balogh B, Millesi H. Are growth alterations a consequence of surgery for prominent ears? *Plast Reconstr Surg* 90:192, 1992.

10

Selected Cartilage-Scoring Otoplasty Techniques

Peter A. Adamson, MD, FRCSC, FACS and
Jason A. Litner, MD, FRCSC

Introduction

In the first half of the 20th Century, cartilage-scoring techniques for otoplasty were used exclusively as an accessory to more aggressive cartilage-cutting techniques. In the early 1960s, a modification of the Luckett procedure was described by Strömbeck[1], in which abrasion of the posterior surface of the auricular cartilage was paired with resection of a portion of the lower antihelix. We have previously mentioned the findings of Gibson and Davis[2] who described bending of cartilage, specifically costal cartilage in their case, away from the side in which the perichondrium was weakened with relaxing incisions, and toward the side having intact perichondrium (**Figure 10-1**). It is interesting that Gibson and Davis were investigating the effect of cartilage scoring in an effort to prevent the troublesome warping of costal cartilage grafts. This observation was later confirmed by Fry[3] with

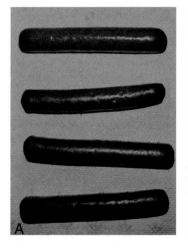
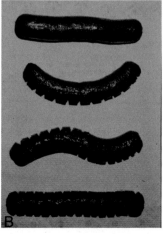

Figure 10-1. The effect of cartilage scoring. (A) Native costal cartilage. (B) Cartilage scoring demonstrating the 'Gibson effect', bending of cartilage away from the scored side.

respect to nasal septal cartilage. These collective observations have since been turned to constructive use in otoplasty.

The theoretical basis for this phenomenon lies in the histologic relationships of the cartilage and perichondrium. The perichondrium consists of a dense connective tissue network that firmly adheres to, and, in fact, merges with the basal layer of chondrocytes on the superficial aspect of the cartilage. The chondrocytes are organized such that they are flattened under some tension at the periphery, in a plane parallel to the surface. The cartilage also contains a matrix composed of densely interwoven elastic fibers that, along with the particular arrangement of the chondrocytes, create interlocked stresses within the cartilage substructure. Thus, when this dense layer is denuded preferentially on one surface, the matrix on that side expands while the stretched layer on the intact side contracts, causing the cartilage to bend as it does. This results from a relative imbalance favoring greater tensile strength on the opposing surface and resulting in cartilage deformation. This unique property furnishes cartilage with its spring or 'memory'.

In 1962, Nordzell[4] noticed this tendency for cartilage to bend eccentrically to the opposite side when abrading one surface of the cartilage itself, rather than just the perichondrium. Others were coming to the same discovery, all at around the same time. In the brief period to follow, a new era of cartilage-scoring otoplasty techniques was ushered in, in Europe and America, by the likes of Cloutier[5], Chongchet[6], Crikelair[7], and Stenström[8]. All of these techniques were similarly based on some type of modification of the superficial layer of the anterior surface of the cartilage, whereas previous techniques had depended on more aggressive modification of the posterior surface.

Cloutier[5] recreated an antihelix by beveling widely along the cut edge of the auricular cartilage. After dividing the cartilage via a posterior approach, Chongchet[6] described making partial thickness parallel longitudinal cartilaginous incisions as well as incisions of the perichondrium over the anterior surface of the proposed antihelix. He preferred wide posterior dissection and suture of the free cartilage edge. Crikelair[7] addressed the cartilage via an anterior skin incision, utilizing a crisscrossing scoring maneuver over the area of the intended antihelix. Stenström[8], conversely, was perhaps the first to report on a technique for blindly 'scratching' the anterior side of the cartilage without dividing it, us-

ing a specially designed instrument known as the Stenström otoabrader. This was introduced through a small medial incision near the cauda helicis to produce an antihelical roll. The degree of scratching of the anterior scaphal surface was adjusted to produce the desired amount of curl. He later modified his technique[9] to include a postauricular incision and wide undermining to expose the scaphal surface, where scoring was completed with his 'scratching instrument'. A marginal excision of a portion of the horizontal helix was suggested as a solution to the problem of persistent upper pole protrusion. He recommended crosswise scratching of the helical tail for cases of continue lobular prominence.

In the decade that followed, a number of modifications were put forward. Davis and Hernandez[10] described a scoring technique via an anterior skin incision at the helical sulcus with sandpapering of the anterior surface of the proposed antihelix. Weerda[11] described a modification of the Converse technique with use of a diamond burr to score the antihelix subperichondrially. Nachlas[12] favored a cartilage-splitting otoplasty that combined use of a diamond burr to abrade the anterior cartilaginous surface. Schufenecker and Reichert[13] modified this scoring technique using a blade with a widely based, superiorly hinged V-Y plasty to lengthen the antihelix. These procedures have been illustrated in greater detail in the chapter dedicated to cartilage cutting techniques (Chapter 9).

Whatever method is used to score the anterior cartilaginous surface, the desired positioning must be stabilized until sufficient inflammatory contracture, and perichondrial fibrosis has occurred to maintain the correction. This can be accomplished via splinting of the ear with appropriate dressings or by combining techniques to include one or more suture methods.

Surgical Technique

The Method of Nordzell

In what is perhaps the single largest known series by a single author, Nordzell[4] reported on his 30-year otoplasty career operating on approximately 870 patients. He used a modified scoring technique in which a postauricular incision through skin and cartilage is carried from the triangular fossa parallel to the helical ridge following the deepest part of the scaphoid fossa all the way to the antitragus (**Figure 10-2**). If the lower part of the ear is protru-

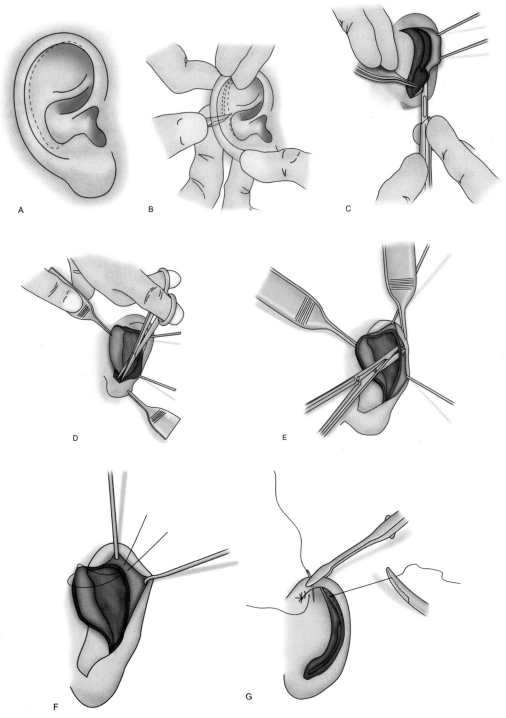

Figure 10-2. The method of Nordzell. (A) Posterior marking from the triangular fossa to the antitragus. (B) Posterior cartilage incision along this line. (C) Elliptical posterior lobule skin excision. (D) Remaining cartilage bridge cut with scissors. (E) Undermining of the lateral cartilage edge by several millimeters. (F) Medial cartilage edge anchored in front of lateral cartilage edge with mattress suture. (G) Skin is closed with a cartilage anchoring suture used for stability.

sive, an elliptical area of retrolobular skin is excised. The cauda helicis is often resected in this scenario, apparently without disadvantage according to the author. This stands in contrast to Webster[14], who judged the tail of the helix to be the key to otoplasty and recommended suturing the tail to the posterior side of the concha. Beernink[15], likewise, emphasized the importance of proper repositioning of the helical tail to properly locate the lower third of the ear.

The anterior skin is then widely undermined and the antihelical cartilage is abraded with a Stryker abrader (Kalamazoo, Mich.) using a rough carbide $1/4$ inch cylinder. Nordzell stresses the importance of abrading the most medial aspect of the antihelix next to the conchal cavity, extending to the triangular fossa. The bending of the cartilage may be seen to happen immediately. Abrasion is continued for roughly 30 seconds until the bend of the lateral part of the antihelical cartilage lays parallel to the line of the lateral cheek. Nordzell finds abrasion superior to other methods because it may be utilized to sculpt the cartilage in a very precise manner. If the concha is enlarged, an elliptical cartilage excision is undertaken at this point. Finally, the lateral antihelical cartilage cut edge is overlapped in front of its opposing edge with Vicryl rapide mattress sutures prior to skin closure. There is no resection of postauricular skin for fear of overcorrecting the middle third and creating a 'telephone ear' deformity.

This method has proved for the author to produce a very reliable correction. In a review of his last 80 consecutive patients, four had small cartilage irregularities, 10 patients were slightly over-corrected or under-corrected by the surgeon's estimation, two had slight asymmetry, and two developed delayed keloids. Three patients were dissatisfied with unsatisfactory correction of the upper part of the ear, requiring revision surgery.

Of interest, the procedure is performed under local anesthesia, even in children. Local infiltration anesthesia is aided by application of a topical anesthetic cream 90 minutes prior to the start of the procedure. In Nordzell's hands, his is a simple procedure that is rapidly and consistently applied, with the correction of each ear taking from 12 to 15 minutes and having a total operative time of about 40 minutes.

The Method of Nolst Trenité

Nolst Trenité's method is a modification of Chongchet's long-practiced scoring technique. Chongchet[5]

utilized a transcartilaginous approach along the lateral side of the proposed antihelix, incising the cartilage and both layers of perichondrium to gain access to the anterior surface of the antihelix. The cartilage spring is then broken and remodeled by parallel longitudinal incisions through perichondrium and the superficial layers of the cartilage. These incisions are made about 1 mm apart under direct visualization.

Precise cartilage bending is, however, difficult to control. Therefore, Nolst Trenité[16] modified the Chongchet technique in several notable ways to achieve more consistent interaural symmetry. First, he undertook subperichondrial rather than supraperichondrial dissection on the anterior surface. He found that this maneuver cut down on postoperative skin discoloration and risk of hematoma. Secondly, he introduced the use of three soluble adjustable mattress sutures (4-0 Vicryl) after subperichondrial anterior scoring was complete. One suture is placed cranially, one centrally, and one caudally. These sutures are placed through the posterior perichondrium traversing the transcartilaginous incision, and are combined with shallower scoring incisions to produce a more predictable remodeling effect. Finally, after cartilage scoring, the remaining cartilage spring is overcome by a horizontal incision at the cauda. Of note, the precise shape of the new antihelix is ascribed to the distance of the mattress sutures in relation to the transcartilaginous incision. Therefore, while Nolst Trenité refers to his method as a modified anterior scoring approach, in essence, this method really qualifies as a combination scoring-suturing-cutting technique.

It is Nolst Trenité's recommendation that the posterior skin excision be planned carefully at least 1 cm medial to the helix and at least 1 cm lateral to the postauricular sulcus to prevent a "glued-on-ear" appearance. Alternatively, a medially based skin flap may be preserved until the conclusion of the case, when the exact amount of redundant skin to be excised can be measured.

Supplementary maneuvers may include excisional reduction of an enlarged concha, or creation of a superior crus or inferior crus by horizontal cartilage incision in these areas. Final tightening of the adjustable mattress sutures, beginning with the central one, is the last maneuver to be completed prior to skin closure with Vicryl rapide. In his review of 65 cases with greater than 1 year and up to 6 years of follow-up, results were satisfactory with few adverse effects. He reported two cases of mildly sharp cartilage edges resulting from too deep a cartilage incision, and two cases of telephone ear from misplaced antihelical sutures.

An important practical consideration for Nolst Trenité that pertains to every surgeon is that the technique applied should not be overly complicated nor overly time consuming. Nolst Trenité prefers this method to others, such as isolated suture techniques, because it can be applied to a greater variety of auricular deformities, especially in ears in which the cartilage is excessively thick or where there is a high concha. In contrast to the Converse technique and its variants, this combination approach is easier to apply and gives less chance of adverse sequelae while offering good long-term results.

The Method of Raunig

Raunig[17] recently reviewed his preferred otoplasty technique, whereby the auricular cartilage is neither sutured nor incised. Raunig's technique relies exclusively on anterior cartilage abrasion and splinting to acquire the desired shaping (**Figure 10-3**). He

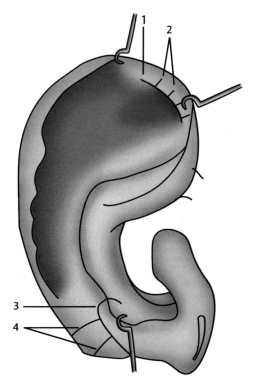

Figure 10-3. The method of Raunig. Antihelical remodeling via an anterior scaphal incision. Radial incisions may be placed in the helical rim to reduce tension. Further incisions in the caudal antihelical margin will allow for shaping in this area.

employs a special diamond-coated electric file for that purpose (Karl Storz and Stuemer, Tuttlingen, Germany). This technique capitalizes on the controlled biomechanical remodeling that occurs when the elastic layer on only one side of the cartilage is disrupted. Raunig prefers use of the diamond-coated file because it provides superlative consistency and smoothness compared with scoring or thinning using a scalpel or comparable instrument.

In his review, Raunig described the use of this technique in 302 ears. Access to the anterior cartilage surface is accomplished via a 10 mm incision concealed in the scapha above the superior crus. The incision is transcartilaginous in this area to allow for further reshaping in the setting of a rigid cartilaginous framework. A subperichondrial tunnel is made along the curve of the desired antihelix down to the level of the antitragus. The diamond-coated file is introduced into this narrow pocket and applied to create a uniform and predictable cartilage thinning until the preferred C-shaped curvature is attained.

Further curvature may be accomplished as necessary by strategic placement of a series of small uniform radial incisions through the helical rim and through the cauda helicis to correct a protruding lobule. Alternatively, two or three cartilaginous wedges may be excised from the groove between the scapha and the helix without disrupting the helical rim. To support scarification of the new antihelix, a posterior subperichondrial tunnel is made along the posterior aspects of the superior crus and the antihelix.

Since this procedure depends solely on cartilage remodeling to make possible the desired improvements, the dressing is especially crucial to the expected result. Raunig places a cotton roll beneath the new antihelix to effect conformation of the roll to the new auricular contour. The helical rim is then taped to the mastoid as a dependable method of retroauricular fixation. A further compressive dressing is removed at 1 week postoperatively. A notable disadvantage of this technique is that additional taping of the ear may be required for up to 8 weeks to maintain the desired alteration, depending on the degree of tension. To avoid this lengthy recuperative period, Raunig has modified his technique to include the use of two subcutaneous mattress sutures for support. One 4-0 PDS or Maxon is placed at the superior crus and a second suture just cranial to the helical tail. In revision cases, Raunig recommends use of permanent sutures.

Significant advantages of this method include decreased incidence of bruising, swelling, and hematoma, preservation of the auricular framework, reduced operating, and recovery time, and absence of foreign body reactivity. As a result, at 4-year follow-up, durable results were achieved while patients experienced few complications. Representative patient examples are shown in **Figures 10-4 to 10-7**. This technique can be applied to most cases of prominent auricles. In extreme cases of conchal excess, a posterior approach may be necessary. However, in this series of 302 ears, cavum resection was required in only four, and sutures were required for stabilization in only 23 cases having excessively rigid concha. Only three ears sustained a loss of correction with two of these necessitating a revision procedure.

The Method of Martin

A recent large series making use of a minimal access anterior scoring technique was published in the UK[18]. In this series, a review is undertaken of Martin's modification of a percutaneous anterior scoring method developed by Mahler[19]. In Martin's modification, a green hypodermic needle is bent and converted into a blade for the purpose of anterior cartilage scoring. Prior to this, local anesthetic containing adrenaline is infiltrated between the cartilage and the subcutaneous tissues along the line of the desired antihelix. In this manner, some hydro-dissection and hemostasis is obtained. The hypodermic needle can be reliably bent into an appropriate scoring instrument by grasping and twisting the needle halfway along the bevel through 90°, thus converting the needle into a fine vertically oriented blade.

The blade, thus modified, is inserted into the existing local anesthetic puncture site and is advanced while infiltrating with the blade parallel to the surface of the cartilage. The scoring action is undertaken while withdrawing the needle, and is repeated as often as necessary to soften the cartilage sufficiently. Care must be taken to avoid repeated scoring over the same point to prevent unwitting full-thickness cutting of the cartilage, which, if present, must be repaired in order to preclude unwanted ridging.

This minimal access-scoring technique is combined with a conservative dumbbell shaped posterior skin excision followed by placement of Mustardé-type permanent sutures to maintain the desired antihelical correction. Martin advocates placement of a double mattress suture that functions as a pulley, enabling exact tension placement.

One advantage of this method is the possibility of using finer suture for this purpose since the cartilage has already been amply weakened to the extent that sutures are used to hold the position rather than to produce it. The use of finer suture under lesser tension may substantially diminish the potential for visible or palpable knots. In this technique, soft tissue dissection and degloving of the auricle is also limited, thus reducing the potential for hematoma, infection, or skin-soft tissue necrosis.

One hundred and fourteen consecutive cases[18] were reviewed using this technique with a mean follow-up of just under 4 years. Excellent and lasting results were obtained with few postoperative complications and high ratings of patient satisfaction. Bleeding occurred in one patient, self-limited infection in four, hypertrophic scarring in two, and recurrence requiring reoperation in one patient. Six patients perceived residual upper pole prominence but only one requested further operative correction. Finally, there was no incidence of hematoma, skin complications, palpable sutures, or cartilage irregularities. The authors attribute the low incidence of complications to the combination of techniques that maximizes the advantages and minimizes the disadvantages of each component part.

The Method of Chait and Nicholson

Chait and Nicholson[20] reported on their extensive experience in 476 patients over 20 years that involved a number of cartilage-manipulating procedures. Their technique begins with a postauricular incision that is crescentic rather than elliptical in shape. The incision should lie approximately 2 cm medial to the rim of the helix. The posterior auricular skin is widely undermined laterally to the posterior edge of the helix. A curvilinear transcartilaginous incision is then extended from the lower border of the antihelix to the superior crus, laying parallel to and about 1 cm from the helical margin. Wide undermining of the anterior skin is undertaken deeply into the concha while the anterior perichondrium is left adherent to the cartilaginous surface.

Scoring of the anterior perichondrium is then performed using parallel longitudinal incisions. If the deformity is limited to an obtuse conchascaphal angle, then scoring is restricted to the perichondrium overlying the scapha. If, on the other hand, the malformation also extends to include a deep concha, then perichondrial scoring is also expanded to include the concha itself. This causes an appropriate
(Text continues on page 79)

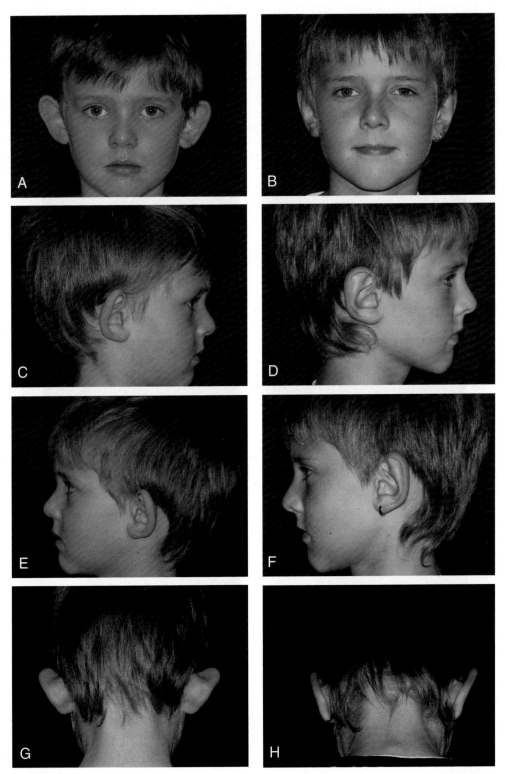

Figure 10-4. (A-D) Preoperative antihelical hypoplasia. (E-H) Three-year postoperative result with the diamond-coated file technique alone. No modeling sutures were used. (*Photos courtesy of Hermann Raunig, MD.*)

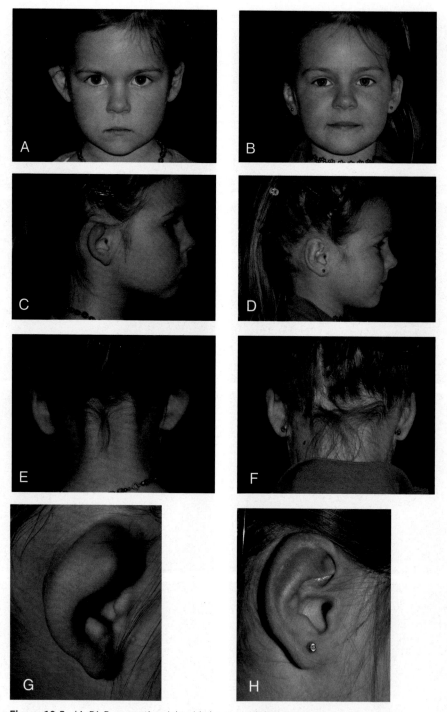

Figure 10-5. (A-D) Preoperative right-sided cup ear deformity. (E-H) Two-year post-operative result with the diamond-coated file technique and reconstruction of the helical rim. No modeling sutures were used. (*Photos courtesy of Hermann Raunig, MD.*)

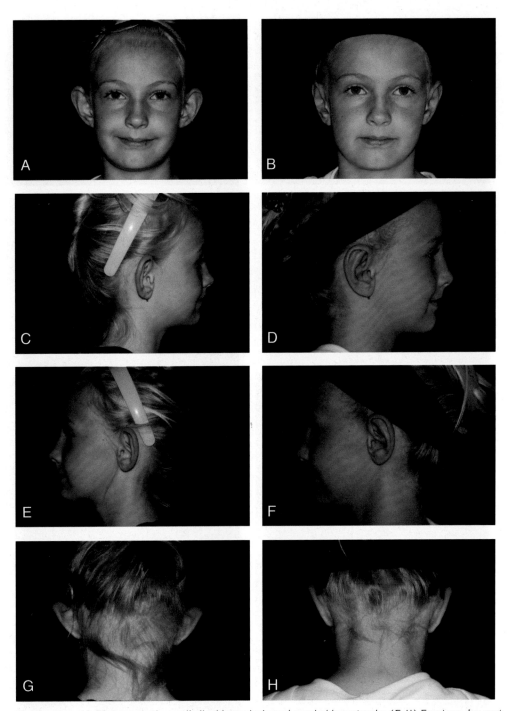

Figure 10-6. (A-D) Preoperative antihelical hypoplasia and conchal hypertrophy. (E-H) Fourteen-day post-operative result with the diamond-coated file technique combined with conchal resection. One absorbable suture was used to preserve the superior crus and two absorbable sutures were used to close the gap after the partial conchal resection. (*Photos courtesy of Hermann Raunig, MD.*)

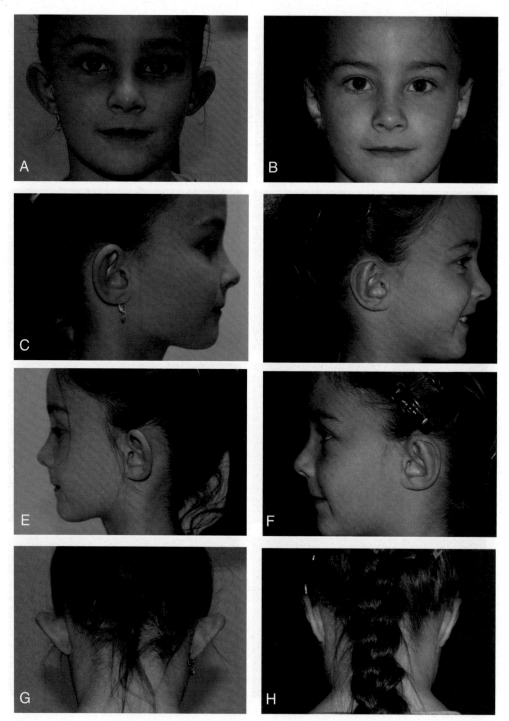

Figure 10-7. (A-D) Preoperative antihelical hypoplasia. (E-H) Four-month postoperative result with the diamond-coated file technique. One absorbable suture was used to fix the superior crus. (*Photos courtesy of Hermann Raunig, MD.*)

degree of folding of the auricular cartilage. A single horizontal mattress suture composed of colorless 4-0 nylon is placed just above the helical tail to hold the desired position. This suture is tightened until the preferred scaphaconchal angle is obtained.

According to the authors, variations of this single technique may be used to treat the two most frequently seen deformities in prominent ears. In the case of a poorly formed antihelix, the scoring recreates an acute cartilaginous roll at the existing antihelix. In the case of a deep conchal bowl, the lateral conchal cartilage is folded into the scapha to assume a new position as the neo-antihelical fold. Excess cartilage may then be trimmed off laterally at the free margin of the transection. An additional advantage is the absence of a redundant skin fold within the concha as is sometimes seen after large conchal resections done from a posterior approach. In addition, the chances for reprotrusion are virtually eliminated because the residual helical rim overlaps the anterior cartilaginous surface.

The Method of Peker and Celiköz

A further modification of Chongchet's anterior scoring technique is one advanced by Peker and Celiköz[21]. In their series of 178 patients treated over an 8-year period, they applied a modified technique involving extensive anterior scoring and posterior rolling of the antihelical cartilage (**Figure 10-8**). As in previously described techniques, a posterior fusiform skin excision is followed by a transcartilaginous incision within the scapha. The anterior cartilaginous surface is scored with a scalpel as described by Chongchet[6]. In cases having a deep concha, anterior dissection and scoring are carried further onto the deepest part of the concha. The free edge of the antihelical cartilage is then rolled over itself posteriorly and secured with 4-0 PDS suture. The skin and perichondrium are closed over this reshaped structure with a running 4-0 catgut suture. Lobule setback is then performed as necessary by suture fixation of the lobular dermis to the periosteum. Finally, the helical root is fixed to the temporoparietal fascia to prevent a telephone ear deformity.

The key advantage of this modification is the increased stability of the antihelical roll that it affords. Rolling the cartilage on itself establishes a natural fold and decreases recurrence rates in comparison to procedures that do not include suture fixation. Additionally, overcorrection of the deformity is not

required since the cartilage alteration remains durable. Corchado[22] agreed that anterior scoring was insufficient for a lasting improvement in thick cartilage and should be supported with permanent sutures.

The Method of Azuara

Azuara[23] reported on a similar technique used in over 100 cases during a 7-year period. A posterior approach is used with resection of a lozenge-shaped area of skin. Care is taken to preserve the postauricular perichondrium and subdermal tissue since maintenance of the antihelical roll depends on suture stabilization through this soft tissue.

Azuara makes his transfixion incision, after marking the cartilage with dye, through the posterior aspect of the cartilage 4 or 5 mm behind the entire length of the future location of maximal prominence of the antihelix. Subperichondrial dissection of the entire anterior aspect of the scapha is undertaken from the fossa triangularis to the antitragus. Multiple multidirectional hemitransfixion (partial thickness) incisions are then made with a no. 15 multi-blade on the anterior aspect of the cartilage at the precise position where the desired antihelix will be formed. This maneuver allows a tension-free posterior rolling of the newly formed antihelical edge. The final step is the placement of two nylon sutures through the preserved posterior perichondrium and soft tissue to further secure the folded cartilage edge. The skin edges are closed with interrupted everting sutures to diminish the risk for a poor scar.

Rubino and colleagues[24] further modified this same technique to incorporate a more extensive anterior dissection to involve the anterior surface of the helix itself. Prevention of a telephone ear deformity is accomplished by supplementary scoring of the helical curvature along the superior third.

Other Notable Scoring Techniques

Many of the early adapters of scoring techniques in otoplasty built on the methods developed by Stenström[8]. An example of a posterior cartilage scoring technique is shown in (**Figure 10-9**). Early significant contributions were made by Staindl[25] and Tolhurst[26]. Tolhurst used specialized instruments via anterior or posterior stab incisions to score the cartilage, though he noted high complication rates. Vecchione[27] advocated needle scoring of the anterior cartilage surface. Ely[28], in Brazil, provided one of the

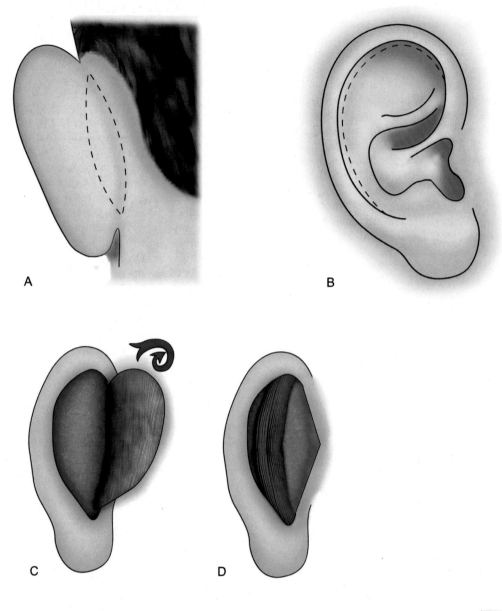

Figure 10-8. The method of Peker and Celikoz. (A) Posterior fusiform skin excision. (B) Cartilage incision within the scapha. (C) Anterior longitudinal scoring of the intended antihelix and concha as necessary. (D) Rolling of the antihelical cartilage posteriorly. (E) Suturing of the tubed cartilage with 4-0 PDS.

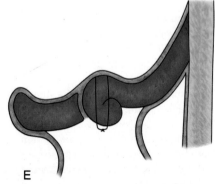

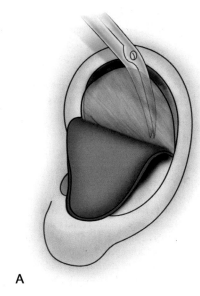
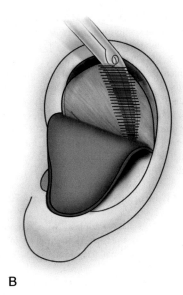

A   B

Figure 10-9. Posterior cartilage scoring technique of Davis. (A) Anterior skin and cartilage are widely incised and undermined. (B) Cartilage is extensively abraded posteriorly with sandpaper down to the helical tail.

first descriptions of small incision otoplasty using a scoring-only technique with a rasp, without the need for skin excision. Nevarre[29] described a novel scoring method using endoscopic carpal tunnel release instruments to correct a flattened antihelix. Tan and colleagues[30] have suggested simple use of an Adson-Brown forceps as their scoring instrument of choice. Di Mascio et al.,[31] preferred use of a dermabrader drill for this purpose in their series of 75 treated ears. Di cio[32] described a technique in 40 patients involving an anterior approach with cartilage abrasion using an electric burr. Rarely, this was combined with conchamastoid mattress sutures when the concha was severely hypertrophied. Outcomes were highly successful and rated by the authors as being safer and more precise than the partial parallel cartilage incision procedure that they had previously favored. Additional techniques including a prominent scoring component tend to combine this with cartilage excision and suture methods. These will be discussed in the chapter dedicated to combination otoplasty methods (Chapter 13).

References

1. Strömbeck JO. Results of surgery for protruding ears. *Acta Chir Scand* 122:138, 1961.
2. Gibson T and Davis WD. The distortion of autogenous cartilage grafts, its cause and prevention. *Br J Plast Surg* 10:257, 1958.
3. Fry HJH. Interlocked stresses in human nasal septal cartilage. *Br J Plast Surg* 19:276, 1966.
4. Nordzell B. Open otoplasty. *Plast Reconstr Surg* 106(7):1466–72, 2000.
5. Cloutier AM. Correction of outstanding ears. *Plast Reconstr Surg* 28:412, 1961.
6. Chongchet V. A method for antihelix reconstruction. *Br J Plast Surg* 16:268, 1963.
7. Ju DM, Li C, Crikelair GF. The surgical correction of protruding ears. *Plast Reconstr Surg* 32:283, 1963.
8. Stenström SJ. A "natural" technique for correction of congenital prominent ears. *Plast Reconstr Surg* 32:509, 1963.
9. Stenström SJ, Heftner J. The Stenström otoplasty. *Clin Plast Surg* 5:465, 1978.
10. Davis JE, Hernandez HH. History of the aesthetic surgery of the ear. *Aesthetic Plast Surg* 2:75–94, 1978.
11. Weerda H. Remarks about otoplasty and avulsion of the auricle (in German). *Laryngol Rhinol* 53:224–57, 1979.
12. Nachlas NE, Duncan D, Trail M. Otoplasty. *Arch Otolaryngol* 91:44, 1970.
13. Schufenecker J, Reichert H. A scoring and V-Y plasty technique. *Facial Plast Surg* 2:119–25, 1985.
14. Webster GV. The tail of the helix as a key to otoplasty. *Plast Reconstr Surg* 44:455, 1969.
15. Beernink JH, Blocksma R, Moore WD. The role of the helical tail in cosmetic otoplasty. *Plast Reconstr Surg* 64:115, 1979.
16. Nolst Trenité GJ. Otoplasty: a modified anterior scoring technique. *Facial Plast Surg* 20(4):277–85, 2004.
17. Raunig H. Antihelix plasty without modeling sutures. *Arch Facial Plast Surg* 7:334–41, 2005.

18. Bulstrode NW, Huang S, Martin DL. Otoplasty by percutaneous anterior scoring. Another twist to the story: a long-term study of 114 patients. *Br J Plast Surg* 56:145–49, 2003.

19. Mahler D. The correction of the prominent ear. *Aesthetic Plast Surg* 10:29–33, 1986.

20. Chait L, Nicholson R. One size fits all: a surgical technique for the correction of all types of prominent ears. *Plast Reconstr Surg* 104(1):190–95, 1999.

21. Peker F, Celiköz B. Otoplasty: anterior scoring and posterior rolling technique in adults. *Aesth Plast Surg* 26:267–73, 2002.

22. Corchado C. A surgical technique for the correction of all types of prominent ears? *Plast Reconstr Surg* 106:948, 2000.

23. Azuara E. Aesthetic otoplasty with remodeling of the antihelix for the correction of the prominent ear: criteria and personal technique. *Arch Facial Plast Surg* 2:57–61, 2000.

24. Rubino C, Farace F, Figus A, Masia DR. Anterior scoring of the upper helical cartilage as a refinement in aesthetic otoplasty. *Aesthetic Plast Surg* 29(2):88–93, 2005.

25. *Staindl O*. Die korrektur der abstehenden ohrmuschel [Correction of prominent ears]. HNO 28:234–40, 1980.

26. Tolhurst DE. The correction of prominent ears. *Br J Plast Surg* 25:261–5, 1972.

27. Vecchione TR. Needle scoring of the anterior surface of the cartilage in otoplasty. *Plast Reconstr Surg* 64(4): 568, 1979.

28. Ely JF. Small incision otoplasty for prominent ears. *Aesthetic Plast Surg* 12:63–9, 1988.

29. Nevarre DR, Maloney C, Wolfort FG. Endoscopic carpal tunnel release instruments used for auricular cartilage scoring and correcting a flattened antihelix. *Plast Reconstr Surg* 106:1214–5, 2000.

30. Tan O, Atik B, Karaca C, Barutcu A. A new instrument as cartilage scorer for otoplasty and septoplasty: Adson-Brown forceps. *Plast Reconstr Surg* 115(2):671–2, 2005.

31. Di Mascio D, Castagnetti F, Baldassarre S. Otoplasty: anterior abrasion of ear cartilage with dermabrader. *Aesthetic Plast Surg* 27(6):466–71, 2003.

32. Di cio D, Castagnetti F, Baldassarre S. Otoplasty: anterior abrasion of ear cartilage with dermabrader. *Aesthetic Plast Surg* 27(6):466–71, 2003.

11

Selected Small Incision and Incisionless Otoplasty Techniques

Peter A. Adamson, MD, FRCSC, FACS and
Jason A. Litner, MD, FRCSC

Introduction

A relatively recent innovation in the world of otoplasty has been the introduction of small incision, endoscopic, and incisionless techniques for the correction of protruding ears. These advances echo the minimally invasive movement that has been pursued elsewhere in surgery. Perhaps the best known of these to date is the incisionless otoplasty technique first promulgated by Fritsch[1] in 1995. Although such techniques have not yet been widely adopted, they are nonetheless highly inventive attempts to improve upon the shortcomings of older modalities.

The key criticism leveled against small incision techniques has been the issue of limited applicability; that is, opponents charge that this technique is relevant only to improvement of the unfolded antihelix and cannot address conchal excess or other auricular abnormalities connected to prominent ears. Moreover, it is alleged that reliance on suture remodeling alone without weakening of the cartilage spring renders these methods more susceptible to relapse. Fritsch[2] has led the way in addressing these limitations by refinement of his technique in subsequent iterations, most recently published in 2004, and described below.

Notwithstanding the criticism of small access techniques, they are not without substantial advantages of their own. The normal auricular structures are retained in their entirety with little potential for contour irregularities or sharp edges. There are no substantive scars and, as a result, no possibility for wound complications such as keloid scarring. Minimal tissue trauma translates to a decreased risk of hematoma and postoperative infection. Lesser undermining also accounts for the lesser degree of postoperative swelling and the presumptively quicker healing. Consequently, prolonged postoperative bandaging is often unnecessary.

Surgical Technique

The Method of Fritsch

The incisionless otoplasty technique has been performed by Fritsch since 1992 and has since undergone several evolutions in technique to permit more expansive treatment of all causal entities in the prominent ear (**Figures 11-1 to 11-17**). The only instruments required are a small single-pronged skin hook, a 21-gauge phlebotomy needle, and 4-0 Mersilene (braided polyester) sutures on cutting needles. Both ears are prepped into the field

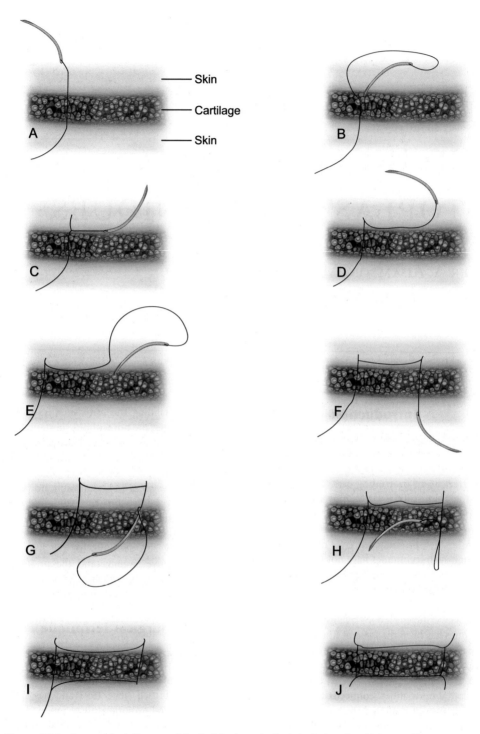

Figure 11-1. A conceptual diagram of the incisionless otoplasty technique in which a continuous, percutaneously introduced suture loop is shown in various stages of placement.

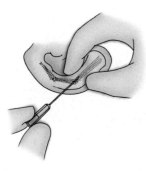

Figure 11-2. A 20-gauge needle is used to weaken the cartilage spring to an almost flaccid condition so that there is a minimal of resistance to the retention sutures.

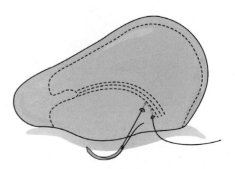

Figure 11-5. Going through-and-through the pinna, the needle exits on the posterior conchal surface. This completes the first "short limb" of the retention suture.

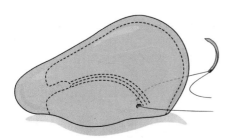

Figure 11-3. The suture loop starts with a through-and-through conchal bowl needle pass.

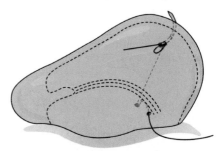

Figure 11-6. The first "long limb" of the retention suture travels subcutaneously on the posterior surface of the pinna and takes bites into the perichondrium in order to stabilize the suture on the cartilage and help prevent bow-stringing.

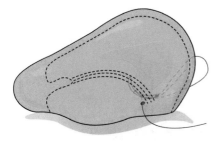

Figure 11-4. The loop then goes through exactly the same anterior exit hole, subcutaneously and to a new skin exit point on the anterior conchal bowl.

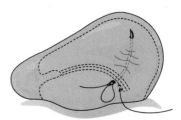

Figure 11-7. The start of the second "short limb" brings the suture to the anterior surface of the pinna.

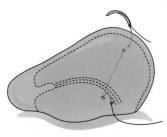

Figure 11-8. The needle and suture are pulled anteriorly and redirected.

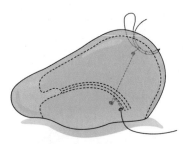

Figure 11-9. Similar to the first "short limb", a subcutaneous route is chosen on the anterior pinna.

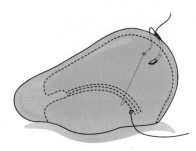

Figure 11-10. A through-and-through placement of the needle redirects the suture to a site that will commence the second "long limb".

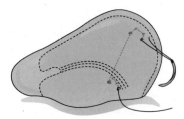

Figure 11-11. The suture returns to the posterior surface completing the second "short limb".

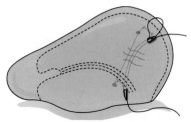

Figure 11-12. The second "long limb" places the suture back to the original entry site and is performed similar to the first "long-limb".

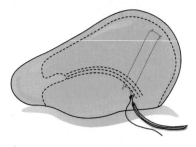

Figure 11-13. The percutaneous suture retention loop is completed.

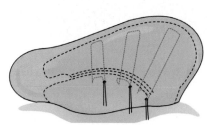

Figure 11-14. Usually, a series of two or three retention sutures is required to hold the neo-antihelix in position. Next, knots are placed in coordination with the contralateral side.

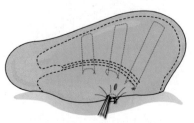

Figure 11-15. A single prong skin hook is used to pull on the elastic skin and submerge the knots below the skin and onto the cartilage.

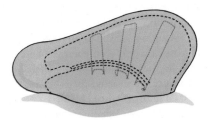

Figure 11-16. The final series of subcutaneous retention sutures holding the ear in position.

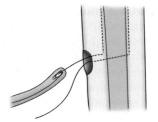

Figure 11-17. A key concept is the right angle placement of the needle and suture from the skin surface to the cartilage area to ensure that the suture loops and knots will submerge without catching on the skin and causing dimpling.

simultaneously using plastic otology drapes. The ears are heavily infiltrated with a vasoconstrictive local anesthetic both circum-aurally and on either side of the pinna at the desired location of the antihelix. This is done with care using a small-gauge needle until blanching is noted. This procedure can be readily performed under local anesthesia alone, although general anesthesia may be required in children.

The area of maximal prominence of the intended antihelical roll can be simulated with bending of the pinna to observe the light reflex and the most natural line of least resistance to deformation. Fritsch notes the futility of this technique in infants as their overly soft cartilage is inclined towards accordion-like folding as opposed to smooth bending when retention stitches are placed.

Fritsch had observed the definite spring-like memory within the auricular structure that tends to defy corrective efforts. If one hopes to obtain a lasting improvement, this cartilage spring must first be weakened and rendered pliable. The addition of methods for breakage of the cartilage spring to the percutaneous suture technique is instructive in that the author believes it essential to lessen the likelihood of relapse. Fritsch's instrument of choice for this function is a phlebotomy needle held as a microknife. The needle is introduced through two to three tiny pinhole incisions on the anterior skin and it is used to produce multiple linear scores spanning the intended line of the antihelical roll. The needle passes are placed partially or, sometimes, completely through the cartilage thickness in as many passes as are needed to completely break the intrinsic cartilage spring. Care is taken to avoid confluence of the needle tunnels to reduce the potential space for accumulation of fluid pockets.

After the cartilage is made sufficiently compliant, retention sutures are placed to maintain stability of the new antihelix. The suture is introduced on the posterior surface of the auricle and is passed perpendicularly through the cartilage and anterior skin in the location revealed by the antihelical bend. Every subsequent pass of the suture is then reintroduced precisely through the exact previous exit point. The single skin hook can be used to expose the entry and exit points and to retract skin adequately to the extent that suture bridges do not occur and that epithelial tissue is not inadvertently dragged subcutaneously into the suture line. The needle is then passed percutaneously through anterior perichondrium and exits through the anterior skin to create the desired width of the transverse arm of the horizontal mattress suture. The needle is then again passed perpendicularly through the cartilage back to the posterior surface and the mattress suture is completed when the needle is passed back through posterior perichondrium to exit exactly via the original entry point. The single-pronged skin hook is used throughout to ensure that the suture has passed appropriately and is not being caught up at all. The knot is then tied, cinched down tightly to achieve the preferred degree of folding, and buried subcutaneously through the needle exit point.

The reentry of the suture through exactly the same puncture site from which it exited at each turn is of critical importance to avoid the occurrence of buried squamous epithelium. Entry of the needle at right angles to the surface discourages dimpling of the skin. Finally, suture 'bites' should be as deep as possible through perichondrium to diminish the risk of suture extrusion, skin erosion, or 'bowstringing' of the thread. Three to four stitches are generally needed per side to achieve adequate correction and slight overcorrection is considered desirable to allow for some postoperative stretch.

Since his original description of the incisionless technique, Fritsch has extended the indications for its use by allowing more comprehensive correction of conchal excess. This is done in the customary manner of postauricular soft tissue excision and placement of a Furnas-type conchamastoid suture, all except that this work is done completely endoscopically. Endoscopic access is via two small stab incisions in the postauricular sulcus. A guarded monopolar needle-tip cautery is utilized to develop a postauricular subcutaneous pocket. With the aid of the endoscope, a forceps is introduced to bluntly remove the requisite postauricular soft tissue. Any bleeding points are vigorously controlled and the incision is extended slightly as necessary for exposure for control of bleeding. The conchal cartilage is not cauterized to prevent injury. Once an adequate tissue bed has been developed, percutaneously placed retention sutures are used to retract the concha posteriorly to create a suitable concha-mastoid angle.

Of note, operative work between the two areas, the mastoid and the antihelix, is isolated so that infection in either area is less liable to extend to involve the entire ear and, specifically, the sutures within the other area. Thus, operative undermining for conchal correction is limited to a pocket overlying the

mastoid to avoid connection with the antihelical area. If endoscopic conchal setback is deemed necessary, it is performed in advance of the antihelical work. Great caution is taken to promote a bloodless field. In most cases, no postoperative bandages are used except in the event of a moist conchal dissection in which case a mastoid-type dressing may be applied for 24 hours (**Figure 11-18**).

A useful aphorism presented by the author is that "patient satisfaction and long-term success occur at the time of surgery". Therefore, he encourages diligent attention to symmetry in every detail. Diligence, though, does not imply that the operation must move excessively slowly and, in fact, the author can throw each percutaneous stitch in about 2 to 3 minutes. The operation, accordingly, confers a cost-benefit in addition to its long-term reliability, low complication rate, and attractiveness to patients. Representative examples of patient results are shown in **Figures 11-19 and 11-20**.

Other Notable Small Access Techniques

The application of small access techniques to otoplasty is not a new concept. Ely[3] put forth the earli-

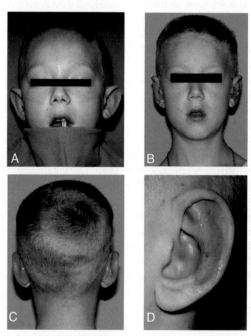

Figure 11-18. Perioperative patient photos showing atraumatic nature of the incisionless technique. (A) Immediate preoperative. (B) Immediate postoperative. (C) One hour postoperative without need for dressing. (D) Close-up of one hour postoperative. (*Photos courtesy of Michael Fritsch, M.D.*)

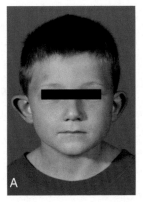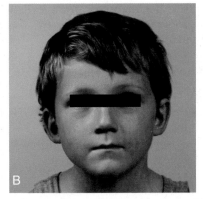

Figure 11-19. Patient results with the incisionless otoplasty technique. (A) Preoperative, and (B) Postoperative. *(Photos courtesy of Michael Fritsch, M.D.)*

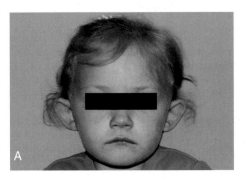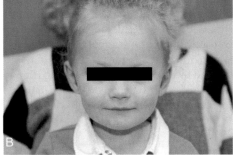

Figure 11-20. Patient results with the incisionless otoplasty technique. (A) Preoperative, and (B) Postoperative. *(Photos courtesy of Michael Fritsch, M.D.)*

est description that we know of more than 20 years ago. He proposed the use of two 0.5 cm incisions to gain access to the lateral surface of the auricular cartilage. By means of these incisions, the cartilage surface may be thinned with a rasp along the desired line of the antihelix. The conchal cartilage may be similarly treated to encourage posterior folding in the setting of an enlarged concha. Skin is not excised in this technique.

The incisionless otoplasty has also been promoted by Merck[4] in Europe, by Peled[5] in Israel, and by Connolly[6] in New Zealand. To our knowledge, these proponents perform the technique in almost, if not exactly, the same way as previously described. Merck began practicing his 'stitch method' in 1995 and began publicizing his experience in 2000, although he has not formally published it in the medical literature so few details are available. He has reported on his website to have performed this

procedure on over 5000 ears. For children younger than 11, Merck chooses to perform the procedure under general anesthesia. In children older than 12 and in adults, local anesthesia is used. Of interest, during the operation every awake patient may not only check but also actually helps to determine the position of their ears using a hand-held mirror. The patient goes home immediately after the operation, without bandages.

Zambudio et al.,[7] attempted to apply a minimally invasive technique in children involving scoring of the anterior surface of the cartilage with a rasp followed by percutaneous placement of mattress sutures through the anterior skin. A good aesthetic result was obtained in all of 22 ears, but not without serious complications. Superficial skin necrosis occurred in three patients, partial loss of correction at the superior pole in four, and sutures were visible through the skin in six patients. The authors justifiably conclude that this complication rate is unacceptably high and warn that sutures be placed from the posterior surface.

We previously mentioned in this chapter the use of an endoscope to assist in the correction of the prominent concha. Graham and Gault[8,9] should be credited with the first description of the endoscopic-assisted otoplasty. Endoscopic techniques first gained acceptance in facial aesthetic surgery, particularly for brow lifts, at around the same time. The authors adapted these techniques for use in otoplasty by introducing the endoscope through scalp incisions. In their technique, the posterior (medial) surface of the cartilage is weakened by abrasion with a custom-made abrader in order to create a new antihelical roll. One or two postauricular stab incisions are used to insert permanent scaphamastoid sutures to secure the desired contour.

It is interesting to note that small access techniques have not gained immense traction in otoplasty just as they have been declining in other areas of facial plastic surgery. Open access techniques are currently enjoying a renaissance as more and more surgeons find that they can better secure and maintain the desired result by removing tissue. Surely, the pendulum of popular opinion will continue to swing through its path and, as it does, it is heartening to see Fritsch and others continue to lead the way in transporting otoplasty techniques into the new millennium.

References

1. Fritsch MH. Incisionless otoplasty. *Laryngoscope* 105 (70):1–11, 1995.
2. Fritsch MH. Incisionless otoplasty. *Facial Plast Surg* 20(4):267–70, 2004.
3. Ely JF. Small incision otoplasty for prominent ears. *Aesthetic Plast Surg* 12(2):63–9, 1988.
4. Merck W. http://www.ear-clinic.com/www/ohren_faden.php
5. Peled IJ. Knifeless otoplasty: how simple can it be? *Aesthetic Plast Surg* 19(3):253–5, 1995.
6. Connolly A, Bartley J. 'External' Mustardé suture technique in otoplasty. *Clin Otolaryngol Allied Sci* 23(2):97–9, 1998.
7. Zambudio G, Ruiz JI, Guirao MJ, Sánchez JM, Girón O, Gutiérrez MA. Anterior approach otoplasty for treatment of prominent ears in children. A minimally invasive technique. *Cir Pediatr* 20(2):119–21, 2007.
8. Graham KE, Gault DT. Endoscopic assisted otoplasty: a preliminary report. *Br J Plast Surg* 50(1):47–57, 1997.
9. Graham KE, Gault DT. Clinical experience of endoscopic otoplasty. *Plast Reconstr Surg* 102(6):2275, 1998.

12

Selected Cartilage-Suturing Otoplasty Techniques

Peter A. Adamson, MD, FRCSC, FACS and
Jason A. Litner, MD, FRCSC

Introduction

We have already described, in chapter 6, our graduated cartilage-sparing otoplasty approach that depends on suture techniques for the majority of its long-term stability. In our hands, this technique has yielded very reliable and enduring results, without exposing the patient to the unnecessary risk of long-term cartilage irregularities[1]. We have not personally experienced significant issues with relapses requiring revision.

Since the original introduction of cartilage-sparing suture techniques by Mustardé[2], numerous authors have adopted these principles almost without modification. Distinct advantages remain to this day owing to the fact that no through and through cartilage incisions are made. In addition, transcartilaginous sutures can be thrown, test-tied, and kept, or redone as desired to achieve a natural antihelical curvature. This is in contrast to the cartilage-cutting techniques reviewed earlier, in which the cartilage incisions are irreversible and uncorrectable. The suture approach is relatively simple to learn and straightforward to teach. It is easily reproduced and requires a more limited dissection and tissue trauma as compared to more aggressive maneuvers. Yet, the classic Mustardé technique has been plagued,

according to some authors[3], by a high rate of suture extrusion and loss of correction. As a result, in the next chapter, we will review some of the significant modifications and adaptations that have incorporated multiple techniques as an eclectic approach in an effort to overcome the failings of each.

Nevertheless, like us, a preponderance of authors continues to hold cartilage-sparing mattress suture techniques in high regard and to practice them dependably (**Figure 12-1 and 12-2**). In this chapter, we will highlight the considerable experiences of these surgeons.

Surgical Technique

The Method of Bull

Bull[4] reported on his otoplasty experience using the Mustardé technique almost exactly as it had been personally described to him. Bull had previously seen many examples of the deficiencies associated with earlier techniques. These had relied too heavily on postauricular skin excision to maintain the medialization and often resulted in a 'pinned down' appearance with obliteration of the postauricular sulcus such that patients had difficulty even in wearing glasses. In his estimation, overreliance

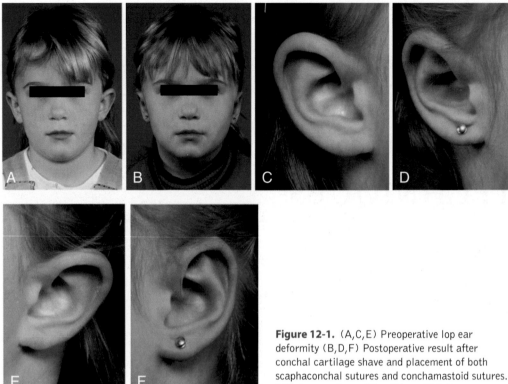

Figure 12-1. (A,C,E) Preoperative lop ear deformity (B,D,F) Postoperative result after conchal cartilage shave and placement of both scaphaconchal sutures and conchamastoid sutures. (*Photos courtesy of Tom Wang, M.D.*)

on reduction of the conchamastoid angle continued in the era of cartilage-incising techniques because these methods did not always give a good correction. Instead, a prominent ear often remained with the achievement only of a 'sharp, tender, and crenulated antihelix'. Subsequent adoption of the techniques of Mustardé, Stenström, and Converse resulted in procedures that consistently produced a formed antihelix but often neglected the conchal cartilage, resulting in ears that were still prominent. Mustardé's understanding of this fact was instrumental to his modification of his own technique that prescribed positioning of the sutures, to roll the antihelical fold anteriorly in such a way, that the conchamastoid angle appeared reduced. This likely occurred by 'borrowing' cartilage from the lateral concha to create the antihelical fold. In his 10-year review of this technique[5], Mustardé encountered satisfying results.

Bull places the postauricular incision in the postauricular fold to keep it far from the transcartilaginous sutures. This is a modification of the original description of an incision located in the midportion of the postauricular curvature of the ear. Despite locating the incision in the sulcus, the cartilage may be easily delivered to allow for appropriate alteration, according to Bull.

The author also subscribes to Mustardé's insistence on use of silk suture material. He prefers a natural 3-0 white silk suture on a reverse cutting needle to any synthetic fiber. Synthetic fibers have a smooth, slippery texture that encourages unraveling when knots are cut closely. On the other hand, long suture ends on the knots risk irritation of the overlying skin and resultant extrusion of the suture. White silk stitches do not show through the skin and may be cut close to the knot without fear of unraveling. In the experience of Bull, they have given way to few problems over 25 years. This stands out against his experience with various monofilament and braided Teflon sutures in which suture infection was commonplace.

Precise placement of the horizontal mattress sutures is crucial to the result and to the avoidance of problems associated with the Mustardé technique. It is vital that the needle enter and exit the cartilage at a right angle, so that it tracks along the perichondrium, taking a sizeable 'bite' without being too close

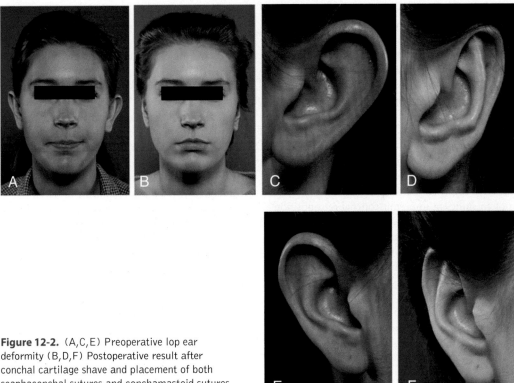

Figure 12-2. (A,C,E) Preoperative lop ear deformity (B,D,F) Postoperative result after conchal cartilage shave and placement of both scaphaconchal sutures and conchamastoid sutures. (*Photos courtesy of Tom Wang, M.D.*)

to the skin. The first suture is placed at the lower pole about 5 mm from the base of the helical tail after the tail has been freed to allow for posterior rolling. It may sometimes be necessary to excise the tail if it is excessively long. Three sutures are routinely placed. The medial aspect of each mattress suture is engaged obliquely to make sure to capture the perichondrium to roll the antihelix naturally. The lateral extent of the suture should be located 7 to 8 mm from the apex of the antihelix. Otherwise, there is the tendency for sutures to pull out. The sutures should be placed close together lest there be crimping. The most apical suture at the superior pole must be located obliquely to recreate a triangular fossa and to prevent a 'straight' antihelical fold.

Bull diverges slightly from the original description when it comes to conchal enlargement. In his hands, Mustardé sutures are sometimes inadequate to achieve the desired amount of anterior rolling of the antihelix to diminish conchal prominence. In this situation, he places a single Furnas-type suture[6] securing the concha to the mastoid periosteum. It may rarely be further necessary to excise conchal cartilage in the event that greater retrodisplacement

is desired as a final step prior to skin closure. Bull prefers at the time of his writing to leave the dressing on for 10 days to "splint" the ears in the immediate postoperative period.

Bull found that his slightly modified Mustardé technique gave him consistently satisfactory results. The most frequently encountered problem was recurrence in about 7% of patients. Because the technique preserves auricular anatomy with minimal scarring, revision is considered feasible without a high level of difficulty.

The Method of Tardy

Tardy also subscribes to a cartilage-repositioning procedure that he first presented in 1969[7] and reviewed in detail in 1996[8]. The horizontal mattress suture antihelix-plasty is the primary mode of repair in this technique, although it is necessary to address thick, inflexible cartilage if present. In this instance, reduction of tension on the horizontal mattress sutures may be advisable by shave excision or thinning of the cartilage with a burr or even incisions through the cartilage to facilitate folding.

A posterior elliptical dumbbell-shaped skin excision is performed at the outset of the procedure. The skin of the postauricular sulcus is preserved; otherwise, flattening of the ear is a risk. The postauricular deep soft tissues and perichondrium are not excised because scarification of this area is central to maintenance of the repair. The postauricular skin is then undermined to the helical margin and to the postauricular sulcus.

A deep conchal bowl, when present, is addressed initially, usually by tangential shave with a scalpel of small disks of cartilage representing the prominent posterior eminences of the auricular cartilage. This is often sufficient to permit conchal retropositioning, thereby obviating the need for conchamastoid sutures. This cartilage excision is intended to be partial thickness. On occasion, a very deep cavum will need to be setback with sutures or, rarely, excision of a semilunar crescent of conchal cartilage.

Once the cavum has been addressed, the new antihelix is created. Temporary marking sutures of 4-0 silk may be placed from an anterior approach to designate the desired location of the posterior mattress sutures. In this way, suture placement may be guided precisely without repeatedly traumatizing the cartilage or staining the skin with ink. Once temporary sutures are in place, 3-0 white braided nylon (Tevdek) horizontal mattress sutures are positioned in sequence in a caudal to cephalic direction through and through the cartilage engaging both perichondrial layers. The anterior skin is palpated to ensure that the needle is not passed too superficially. Sutures are placed away from the incision site to prevent suture exposure. Once the antihelix has been suitably folded, the sutures are tied down sequentially. Tardy normally makes use of four or more mattress sutures to evenly distribute tension. Suture overcorrection is unwarranted if their placement is accurate because slippage should be negligible. If lobular prominence persists, it is dealt with at this point. Generally, simple skin excision will be adequate in most cases, although maneuvers that are more aggressive may be justified. A conforming dressing followed by a bulky head dressing is applied and replaced with a smaller dressing for an additional 36 to 72 hours.

Other Notable Suture Techniques

Enthusiasm for anteriorly placed temporary Kaye-type sutures is shared by others[9,10]. These authors concur that temporary sutures help guide proper placement of the permanent antihelical mattress sutures, while minimizing tissue trauma and decreasing operating time.

Multiple large patient series have been reported by proponents of cartilage suture techniques and their derivatives. Koch et al.,[11] investigated their results in 340 patients treated with a modified Mustardé technique. The postoperative outcome was judged to be satisfactory in 91.4% of cases by patients and in 84.7% by the surgeon. Relapse occurred in 17% of patients and was attributed to the intermittent use of absorbable sutures for maintenance of the antihelix. In some cases, this amounted to a slight asymmetry not requiring revision.

Dechamboux et al.,[12] reported their results in 368 patients over the age of 8 years operated on under local anesthesia using a modified suture method. In their technique, conchal malposition was corrected via a posterior approach using conchamastoid sutures, while antihelical unfurling was treated through an anterior approach by scaphal mattress sutures and occasional scoring of the cartilage. A retrospective study showed that 83% of the patients were deemed to have good or very good results. The morbidity rate was low and comparable to other studies.

A nearly identical procedure has been employed by Vital and Printza[13] in Greece. In their review of 86 consecutively treated patients, they presented a modified cartilage-sparing technique comprising of scapha-conchal sutures to recreate an antihelix, conchal setback, and cartilage weakening as necessary by superficial scoring of the medial surface, accompanied by tangential shave of the posterior eminences of the conchal bowl. They recorded good long-term findings with natural-appearing ears and few complications. Occasional cases of relapse were easily corrected by revisional surgery.

A classical cartilage-sparing suture technique was reviewed objectively using McDowell's anatomic criteria. In total, 117 ears in 62 patients were operated on by Vuyk et al.[14] over a 4-year period. The operation was determined to be successful in 108 ears. Recurrence of the preexisting deformity was seen in six ears and overcorrection was noted in three, obliging reoperation in two ears. The most common complication, although considered minor, was suture extrusion, noted in 15 ears. These were treated readily by suture removal in 14. It was concluded that extrusion appeared to be somewhat dependent on the choice of suture material and the location of the knots.

Attwood and Evans[15] also examined their experience with the classic Mustardé technique performed under local anesthesia in 52 patients aged 9 and older. Their analysis revealed a 100% patient satisfaction rate complemented by a low rate of complications. The most frequent complication was superficial infection that was noted in two ears.

Ellis and Keohane[16] have expressed an appeal for a modified Mustardé method that incorporates other elements including conchal setback as well as modification of the lobule. In their experience, this cartilage-sparing modality is simple to use and provides safe and predictable results. This has not been the case for Grassi and Domenici[17] who had noted frequently that dependence on Mustardé-type mattress sutures alone often led to an incomplete result and not infrequent recurrences. In an effort to achieve a more lasting correction, they have expanded their technique in recent years to include superficial scratching of the anterior cartilage surface in the manner of Stenström. In their hands, this modification has yielded more reliably favorable results.

A final technique worthy of mention here is that of perichondrioplasty (**Figure 12-3**). Although not technically a cartilage-suturing maneuver, this procedure does depend on shaping and positioning of the cartilage to produce the desired antihelical fold. In this case, the cartilage is gently folded by excision,

mobilization, and suturing of the posterior perichondrium to draw the antihelical cartilage into a pleasing position. This model depends on the neochondrogenic potential of the perichondrium first demonstrated in experimental studies on the 'cauliflower' ear. The mobilized perichondrium is stimulated to produce new cartilage posteriorly in the area of the newly folded conchoscaphal angle, which, in turn, is designed to maintain the preferred contour. In 1980, Ohlsén and Vedung[18] reported on a modification of their original technique, which was found to give frequent recurrences. In a follow-up of ears treated with the modified technique, a low recurrence rate of only 3.7% was observed.

In this chapter, we have reviewed those series in which a suture-based cartilage-sparing approach much as our own was used as the cornerstone of the authors' preferred otoplasty method. While these techniques have produced favorable results, many authors still choose to combine these techniques with scoring and incision-excision maneuvers in an attempt to realize the best possible and most predictable long-term otoplasty outcomes. In the next chapter, we will call attention to the foremost combination otoplasty techniques to see if, indeed, a blending of methods really does result in superior outcomes.

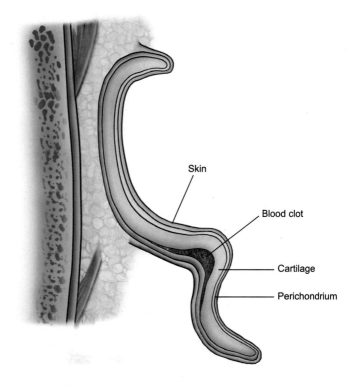

Figure 12-3. Perichondroplasty. A small portion of posterior skin and perichondrium underlying the proposed antihelical line is excised and oversewn. This draws the antihelical cartilage into the desired contour. A blood clot within this potential space fibroses and helps to maintain the new position.

Skin

Blood clot

Cartilage

Perichondrium

References

1. Adamson PA, McGraw BL, and Tropper GJ. Otoplasty: critical review of clinical results. *Laryngoscope* 101(8):883, 1991.
2. Mustardé JC. The correction of prominent ears using simple mattress sutures. *Br J Plast Surg* 16:170, 1963.
3. Horlock N, Misra A, Gault DT. The postauricular fascial flap as an adjunct to Mustardé and Furnas-type otoplasty. *Plast Reconstr Surg* 108(6):1487–90, 2001.
4. Bull TR. Otoplasty: Mustardé technique. *Facial Plast Surg* 10(3):267–76, 1994.
5. Mustardé JC. The treatment of prominent ears by buried mattress sutures: a ten year survey. *Plast Reconstr Surg* 39:382–86, 1967.
6. Furnas DW. Correction of prominent ears by conchamastoid sutures. *Plast Reconstr Surg* 42:189, 1968.
7. Tardy ME Jr, Tenta LT, Pastorek NJ. Mattress suture otoplasty: indications and limitations. *Laryngoscope* 79(5):961–8, 1969.
8. Kotler HS, Tardy ME. Reconstruction of the outstanding ear (otoplasty). In: Ballenger JJ, Snow JB, ed. *Otorhinolaryngology head and neck surgery.* 15th edition. Baltimore: Williams and Wilkins; 1996. p. 989–1002.
9. De la Torre J, Tenenhaus M, Douglas BK, Swinburne JK. A simplified technique of otoplasty: the temporary Kaye suture. *Ann Plast Surg* 41(1):94–6, 1998.
10. Hilger P, Khosh MM, Nishioka G, Larrabee WF. Modification of the Mustardé otoplasty technique using temporary contouring sutures. *Plast Reconstr Surg* 100(6):1585–6, 1997.
11. Koch A, Andes C, Federspil P. Otoplasty: results of a modified form of Mustardé's method. *Rev Laryngol Otol Rhinol (Bord)* 112(3):249–53, 1991.
12. Dechamboux J, Sadek H, Raphaël B. Prominent ears: a simple ambulatory technique under local anesthetic. *Rev Stomatol Chir Maxillofac* 101(6):319–24, 2000.
13. Vital V, Printza A. Cartilage-sparing otoplasty: our experience. *J Laryngol Otol* 116(9):682–5, 2002.
14. Vuyk HD, van der Baan S, Olde Kalter PH. Correction of the external ear using cartilage-sparing techniques. *Ned Tijdschr Geneeskd* 138(13):664–9, 1994.
15. Attwood AI, Evans DM. Correction of prominent ears using Mustardé's technique: an out-patient procedure under local anaesthetic in children and adults. *Br J Plast Surg* 38(2):252–8, 1985.
16. Ellis DA, Keohane JD. A simplified approach to otoplasty. *J Otolaryngol* 21(1):66–9, 1992.16.
17. Grassi C, Domenici R. The surgical remodeling of prominent ears. *Pediatr Med Chir* 18(3):311–3, 1996.
18. Ohlsén L, Vedung S. Reconstructing the antihelix of protruding ears by perichondrioplasty: a modified technique. *Plast Reconstr Surg* 65(6):753–62, 1980.

13

SELECTED COMBINATION OTOPLASTY TECHNIQUES

PETER A. ADAMSON, MD, FRCSC, FACS AND
JASON A. LITNER, MD, FRCSC

Introduction

In the 1950s and 1960s, important strides were made in otoplasty technique. Three fundamental techniques described by Mustardé[1], Stenström[2], and Converse[3] emerged as the representative leaders in the field for the cartilage-suturing, cartilage-scoring, and cartilage-cutting schools of thought, respectively. These techniques rapidly gained popularity; however, over time, many proponents of all three of these had come to notice some occasionally disappointing operative results.

The main shortfalls of these techniques are re-protrusion in the Mustardé otoplasty, poor control of symmetry in the Stenström otoplasty, and visibly sharp edges in the Converse otoplasty. The appearance of a visibly 'operated ear' using cutting techniques was seen to spur greater interest for a time in a classic cartilage-suturing technique. In recent years, concern with isolated cartilage-sparing techniques has focused on the alarmingly high reported rate of loss of correction in some series, at times approaching 25%, and on the very real threat of stitch extrusion (as high as 15%)[4]. Horlock et al.,[4] as a result, recommended routine use of a postauricular fascial flap in suture-dependent otoplasties for subcutaneous knot coverage to successfully decrease the incidence of long-term suture exposure.

Innumerable modifications have since been advanced in pursuit of the 'holy grail' of otoplasty techniques, although the sheer number of methods available attests to the fact that no such panacea yet exists. Many authors now incorporate an eclectic mix of techniques, capitalizing on the benefits of each to create a natural auricular contour. We will characterize several combination techniques in this chapter that are particularly versatile, simply applied, and clearly taught.

Surgical Technique

The Method of Stucker

Stucker first described his combined mattress suture and lateral conchal cartilage resection technique in 1977[5], and he has employed it reliably in over 300 patients[6,7]. His method begins with a fusiform postauricular skin excision that is estimated by rolling the pinna posteriorly over a finger to simulate the desired antihelical fold. The presumed redundant skin is then excised in a subdermal plane followed by separation of the cauda helicis from the lateral conchal cartilage. Often, spreading action of the scissors is sufficient to separate these planes although they may need to be sharply divided. This maneuver preserves the natural roll of the cauda helix as the antihelix is tubed.

Stucker then proceeds with some degree of lateral conchal resection in most patients. Again, the amount of cartilage to be removed is estimated by digitally rolling the antihelix posteriorly. Enough conchal cartilage is excised to allow the mid-portion of the helix to set back after formation of the antihelical fold. A conservative crescent-shaped area of cartilage is removed parallel to the line created by separation of the concha from the cauda helicis. The anterior perichondrium is preserved.

Following lateral conchal cartilage resection, the antihelical relief is created using a classic Mustardé suture technique. Stucker expressly avoids braided sutures because of their propensity for sawing through the cartilage. Instead, three or four 4-0 nylon sutures are used to recreate the desired contour. The preferred location of the mattress sutures may be marked prior to placement using a Keith needle dipped in methylene blue; however, this step may be eliminated when one has become rather facile with the technique. The sutures are tied down sequentially when all are in place. Finally, the skin is closed with a running 4-0 chromic stitch.

Stucker stresses several purported advantages of the technique. First, lateral conchal resection provides for a smooth antihelical transition once the mattress sutures are positioned. Second, a telephone ear deformity is all but averted by preventing excessive projection of the upper and lower poles owing to the resected conchal cartilage. Finally, there is no need for conchamastoid sutures that may predispose to meatal stenosis. In Stucker's long experience with this method, complications were noted to occur in fewer than 3% of patients. A telephone survey revealed that most patients were very satisfied with the perception, symmetry, and appearance of their ears after surgery.

The Method of Farrior

Farrior first published his combination technique in 1959[8] and it has been used faithfully in both his and his son's practice since that time. The Farrior otoplasty combines elements of cartilage sculpting, suturing, and conchal setback techniques using a graduated approach. Although this technique combines a number of maneuvers, they are applied on a case-by-case basis after careful analysis so that only those procedures necessary to achieve the desired result are performed.

As part of this graduated approach, as with ours, the simplest methods are tried first, followed by more complicated maneuvers, as dictated by the particular aberrant anatomy. A problem-specific approach is proposed. Factors considered important in surgical planning are the cartilage thickness and resilience, the depth and degree of conchal cupping, the existing antihelical convexity, the development of the helical rim, the pillar effect of the inferior crus, and the possibility of a resistant superior quarter of the ear[9].

Mattress sutures of 4-0 Mersilene may be used alone in a weak or absent antihelical fold, although Farrior and colleagues most often find it necessary to add scoring of the cartilage to break the resilient spring. In the setting of a deep concha, an elliptical excision is completed with or without the addition of conchamastoid sutures. All maneuvers are accomplished from a posterior approach. A postauricular dumbbell-shaped skin excision and excision of the cauda helicis are regular constituents of the technique. When the upper pole is very resilient, Farrior recommends extending the scaphal scoring incisions superiorly or the conchal rim incision inferiorly into the inferior crus when the intercrural junction is particularly tenacious. Horizontal mattress sutures may be added in the area of the superior crus. If the anterior inferior crus is responsible for a strong pillar effect, then sectioning or removal of a portion of this structure is warranted.

In 2007, Scharer et al.[10] reported on the results of the Farrior otoplasty technique in 75 patients over a 15-year period. The majority of patients (47) underwent conchal reduction, cartilage scoring and mattress suture placement. Twelve underwent conchal setback with sutures alone, 10 had isolated antihelical cartilage scoring with sutures, while grafting and suturing of the superior helical rim was performed in four patients, and two patients had other modifications performed.

Mean follow-up was just over 1 year with generally positive outcomes noted by patients. There were no major complications noted. However, minor complications were surprisingly common with 40 such problems observed in 29 patients. The two most frequently noted complications were suture extrusion and reprotrusion of the superior pole, occurring in 19% and 23% of cases, respectively. The average time to suture extrusion was 15 months, and these instances were relatively easily treated by suture removal in the office without consequence. Despite the high rate of minor complications, the overwhelming majority of patients contacted seemed happy with their results and only 11 patients required minor revision procedures. This led Farrior to conclude, as have others[11,12], that some degree of reprotrusion, particularly at the superior pole, is almost to be expected after otoplasty. The incidence of minor complications noted serves to underscore the difficulties inherent in otoplasty. Representative examples of patient results with the Farrior otoplasty are shown in **Figures 13-1 to 13-3**.

The Method of Caouette-Laberge

In another impressively large series of 500 consecutive cases, Caouette-Laberge et al.,[13] reviewed their experience with a cartilage cutting and anterior scoring otoplasty approach at a single institution over a 12-year span. This technique mirrors the principles of Crikelair and Cosman[14] with some modifications (**Figure 13-4**). Their approach uses a postauricular 3.5 cm incision located 1 cm from the helical margin, so that it will eventually lay hidden in the concavity created by the neo-antihelix. Unlike

in many other techniques, no skin is excised. Very little posterior skin undermining is necessary as the skin incision lies close to the proposed transcartilaginous incision. Limitation of skin undermining discourages hematoma formation and potential devascularization.

A curvilinear cartilaginous incision is made from the cleft between the tail of the helix and the concha parallel to the helical border completely around its circumference into the upper pole. This provides complete access to the anterior surface of the concha, which is widely undermined subperichondrially over the antihelix with a periosteal elevator. Only modest exposure of the conchal cartilage is necessary, as there is frequently no reduction needed here. The transcartilaginous incision is undertaken in this manner so that the origin of the helix is sharply

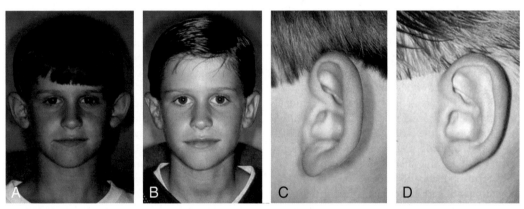

Figure 13-1. (A,C) Preoperative antihelical hypoplasia. (B,D) Postoperative result. (*Photos courtesy of Edward Farrior, M.D.*)

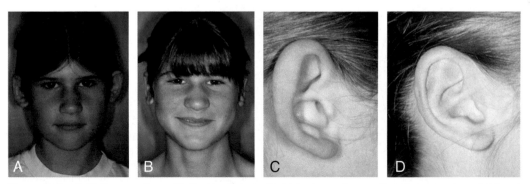

Figure 13-2. (A,C) Preoperative antihelical hypoplasia. (B,D) Postoperative result. (*Photos courtesy of Edward Farrior, M.D.*)

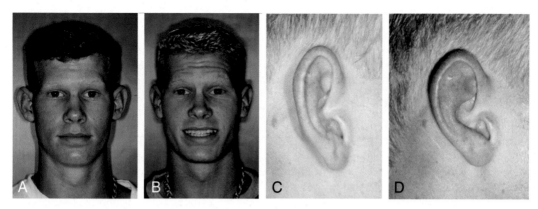

Figure 13-3. (A,C) Preoperative antihelical hypoplasia. (B,D) Postoperative result. (*Photos courtesy of Edward Farrior, M.D.*)

sectioned. Thus, the helical cartilage becomes like a "handle" that can follow the posterior rotation of the antihelical fold as it is formed. This incision is intended to prevent the helix from springing back and reprotruding at the superior pole. It is important to maintain a uniform helical rim segment that is not too wide, as it will tend to protrude, and not too narrow, as it will tend towards unnatural bowing.

Once anterior access is obtained, bi-directional partial thickness scoring incisions are made in the anterior aspect of the cartilage to recreate a normal fan-shaped antihelix that curves both superiorly and posteriorly. The inferior extent of these incisions forms the lateral border of the concha. The incision here is carried through the full thickness of the cartilage to produce a normally sharp fold in

this area. With this incision, the surgeon is able to set the appropriate conchal height. Since this collection of incisions will have overcome the intrinsic elastic memory, the cartilage should maintain its new position without the help of sutures. The sharp bend of the concha is ensured with two sutures of 5-0 plain gut that are utilized to ensure a smooth cartilaginous folding.

Occasionally, it is necessary to expose and lower the projection of the antitragus. Finally, in most cases, lobular prominence must be treated by fixation of the cauda helicis to the adjacent posterior concha after limited undermining of both structures. These can be suitably apposed with a simple 5-0 plain gut suture. Rarely, a longer-acting suture material such as a 5-0 Maxon is used in constricted

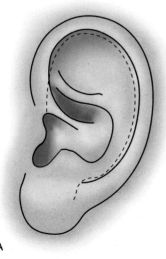

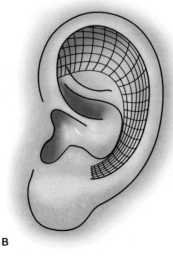

Figure 13-4. The method of Caouette-Laberge. (A) Location of the posterior cartilage incision as seen from the front view (B) Orientation of the partial-thickness anterior cartilage scoring incisions.

A

B

ears with a small helical circumference. Since this technique produces a complete disjunction between the helix and the antihelix, it is crucial to maintain correct positioning during redrapage and dressing placement to avert anterior or posterior luxation of the helix.

A significant point raised by the authors is the likelihood of elevation of the upper helical cartilage when a prominent lobule is set back. This owes to the fact that the entire structure is in continuity, so lowering of one end will lead to an elevation of the other end. In an effort to prevent this effect, the helical continuity must be interrupted by a 2 to 3 mm wedge resection just above the cauda helicis. This will permit posterior positioning of the lobule without movement of the helix itself. In the authors' experience, any apparent skin excess rapidly flattens with scar contraction. They make a point of discouraging skin excision because any reliance on skin to retrodisplace the ear as opposed to adequate destabilization of the cartilage will predispose to long-term failure. This position is shared by Sénéchal and Chauffeté[15]. There is no need for overcorrection because partial relapse caused by stretch is not expected as it is with a suture technique. The authors leave a closed dressing for the first week. They do not believe this to be detrimental, following the counsel of Elliot[16] that unusual pain and/or bleeding are always the harbinger of an early postoperative hematoma or pressure-induced complication.

In their chart review of 500 consecutive cases performed using this technique, the authors evaluated both short-term and long-term complications. Early problems included bleeding in 2.6%, hematoma in 0.4%, mild anterior skin ulceration in 0.6%, and wound dehiscence in 0.2% of patients. All minor wounds healed spontaneously. There were no cases of infection or skin necrosis. The most frequently seen late complications included asymmetry in 5.6% and residual deformity in 4.4% of cases. Secondary surgery was performed in 1.2% of patients for the above reasons. Other noted complications included keloid scars in 0.4% and inclusion cysts in 0.6% of patients.

A questionnaire was also sent to patients at least 2 years after surgery to elicit any ongoing issues they may have had with their ears. A high response rate was obtained. Reports such as these are highly valuable and instructive as long-term patient assessments are difficult to find for this procedure. The subjective problems noted by patients were not insubstantial. Residual pain was reported by 5.7%, persistent hypesthesia by 3.9%, cutaneous reactions such as eczema and intertrigo by 9.8% of patients, abnormal scarring by 1.5%, and sensitivity to cold or touch by 7.5%. Moreover, a sizeable percentage (18.4%) described asymmetry of auricular contour and 4.4% reported an abnormal shape. Nevertheless, 94.8% of patients stated that they were satisfied or very satisfied with the results of their surgery. Of those unhappy with their outcomes, 4.2% were dissatisfied while only 1% reported being very dissatisfied.

Of interest, when these complications were analyzed for possible causal factors, a two-surgeon team was found to be the most significant contributor. In these cases, one ear was operated upon by the senior surgeon while the other ear was operated upon by a resident surgeon. This arrangement resulted in a more than 3-fold incidence of late deformities, indicating a considerable learning curve associated with this surgery.

Overall, complications in this large series compared favorably with other reports, with a remarkably low infection rate even without the use of antibiotic prophylaxis. This lowered risk may be because no permanent suture material is used. Of note, suture extrusion and fistulae are not a risk of this procedure. Additionally, keloid formation was decidedly infrequent, perhaps owing to the lack of skin excision and resultant tension on the wound closure.

The Method of Spira

Spira[17] has used a modification of the classic Mustardé technique[1] to set back protruding ears in more than 200 cases over 30 years (**Figure 13-5**). The ear is marked prior to infiltration of local anesthesia using a 30-gauge needle that has been lightly abraded using a scratch pad to remove its silicone coating. First, rows of ink marks are placed on the ear's anterior surface after lightly folding the scapha. The first row of marks follows from the superolateral aspect of the superior crus down to the scapha above the helical tail. Two marks are placed within the fossa triangularis for placement of sutures in this area. A second row of ink marks, representing the inferior placement of the antihelical mattress sutures, is located just medial to the reformed antihelix within the lateral concha. Finally, a third row of marks just medial to the line described above denotes the desired position of the conchal sutures for conchal medialization. The ink marks are transposed to the cartilage and posterior skin surface by passing the

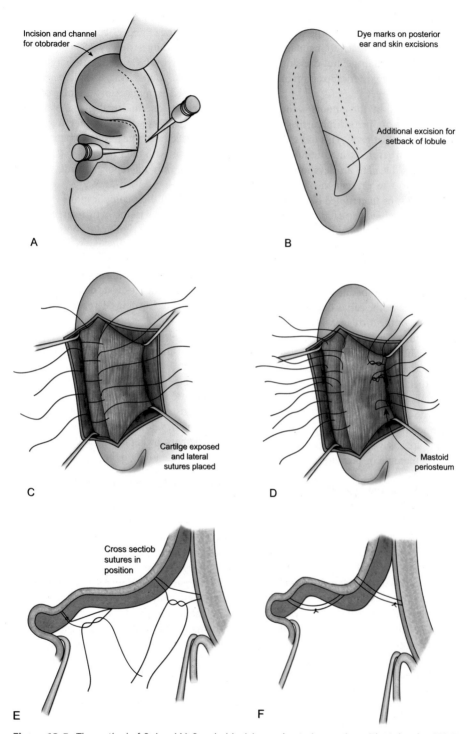

Figure 13-5. The method of Spira. (A) Scaphal incision and anterior scoring with otobrader. (B) Posterior marking and lobular skin excision as needed. (C) Placement of scaphaconchal sutures. (D) Placement of conchamastoid sutures. (E) Cross-section of sutures in position. (F) Conchal sutures tied down first. *(Continued)*

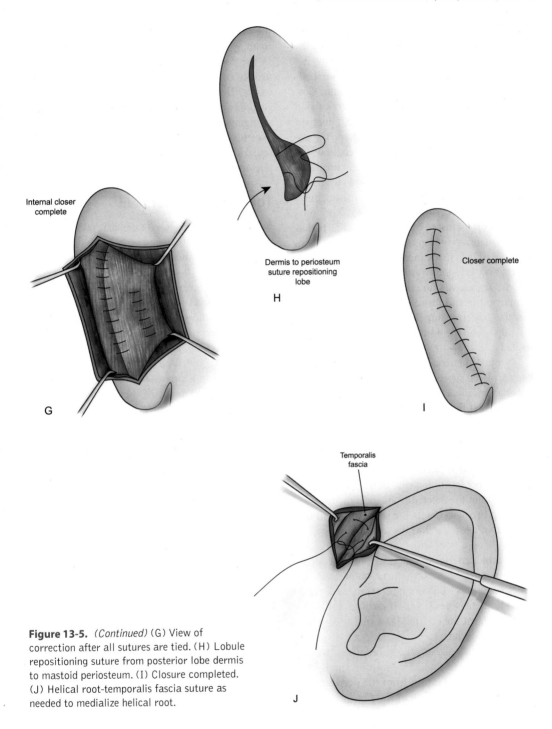

Figure 13-5. *(Continued)* (G) View of correction after all sutures are tied. (H) Lobule repositioning suture from posterior lobe dermis to mastoid periosteum. (I) Closure completed. (J) Helical root-temporalis fascia suture as needed to medialize helical root.

needle through the previously drawn marks anteriorly and wetting the distal end and shaft of the needle with methylene blue before withdrawing it.

A small 3 mm incision is made within the shadow of the helix at the superior crus. A Freer or Cottle elevator is used to undermine the anterior skin over the site of the intended antihelix. A Dingman otobrader is then used to cautiously abrade the anterior cartilage surface over the entire length of the proposed antihelix. Failure to adequately break the cartilaginous spring may incline towards relapse in the late postoperative period. For this reason, Spira now applies this scoring maneuver to every otoplasty rather than just to older patients as he had in the past. Attention is then turned posteriorly where a linear incision is made incorporating only a small elliptical skin excision overlying the posterior lobule. More aggressive skin excision is not planned as a component of this procedure. The skin overlying the entire posterior auricle and mastoid is widely undermined and the postauricular muscle is bluntly retracted.

Horizontal mattress sutures of 4-0 white Mersilene are placed superiorly to inferiorly in sufficient number (typically a minimum of four sutures) to accomplish antihelical folding. Next, at least two conchamastoid sutures are placed to affix the concha to the mastoid periosteum. Conchal sutures are tied down prior to antihelical sutures to avoid overtightening of the antihelix. Employment of fewer sutures in either location is one factor predisposing to recurrence of the deformity. In addition, use of a noncutting needle prevents the small breaks in the cartilage that allow for sutures to tear through. In cases involving a very large concha, care must be taken to avoid anterior displacement of the concha by these sutures with consequent obliteration of the meatus. In this situation, it is preferable to cut a 1 cm wide laterally based flap of cartilage and perichondrium from the conchal floor that is then sutured to the mastoid.

Attention is finally turned to adjuvant procedures as needed. The lobule, if protruberant, is corrected using a single suture from the deep dermis to the most inferior portion of the concha. If there is outward angulation of the helical root superiorly, it is treated with a helical root-deep temporalis fascia mattress suture that is placed through a 4 mm incision located at helical sulcus. All incisions are closed with 4-0 chromic gut after antimicrobial irrigation. Since there is no skin excision, care must be taken to assiduously reapproximate the edges of

the redundant skin. As is our protocol, Spira prefers treating the patient with perioperative antibiotics. In the postoperative period, the postauricular skin usually conforms to the new sulcus within several weeks. This process is to be preferred to a skin excision as it is designed to prevent long-term bowstringing of the sutures. Spira has demonstrated over his long otoplasty career that his 'cookbook' setback otoplasty yields consistently favorable late postoperative results.

The Method of Burstein

Burstein initially had used a conchal 'take-out' technique[18] for years but, based on his cumulative experience, he made numerous modifications and later reported on his 10-year experience with his current technique[19] (**Figure 13-6**). As with Spira, methylene blue is used on a 22-gauge needle to mark the desired antihelical fold, superior crus, and conchal borders. The posterior and anterior skin is infiltrated with local anesthetic but a vasoconstrictive agent is avoided on the anterior surface. An S-shaped incision is carried out on the posterior skin from the highest point of the proposed antihelix down to the lobule. A microcautery needle is used to dissect subcutaneously to the helical rim and over the mastoid periosteum.

The scapha is then pierced posteriorly just below the helical rim at the level of the superior crus. A narrow subcutaneous anterior tunnel is created and an otoabrader is introduced to make multiple microabrasions of the perichondrium and cartilage along the course of the superior crus and antihelix. In younger patients with very pliable cartilage, undermining with scissors and a dissector may be enough to weaken the cartilage without the need for further scoring. It is important not to transect the scapha with this maneuver. Limited skin undermining is advocated on the anterior scapha to avoid a potential hematoma.

Following anterior abrasion of the cartilage, 4-0 clear nylon mattress sutures are placed to create the proposed antihelical line and superior crus. In order to determine the precise location of these sutures, a caliper is used to measure 6 mm on either side of the center of the tattoo marks. Reasonably small bites are taken to prevent cartilage bunching. Placement of four sutures in this manner produces an antihelical fold of a predictable height above the plane of the scapha. The sutures can be adjusted to achieve an antihelical height that is slightly lower than the

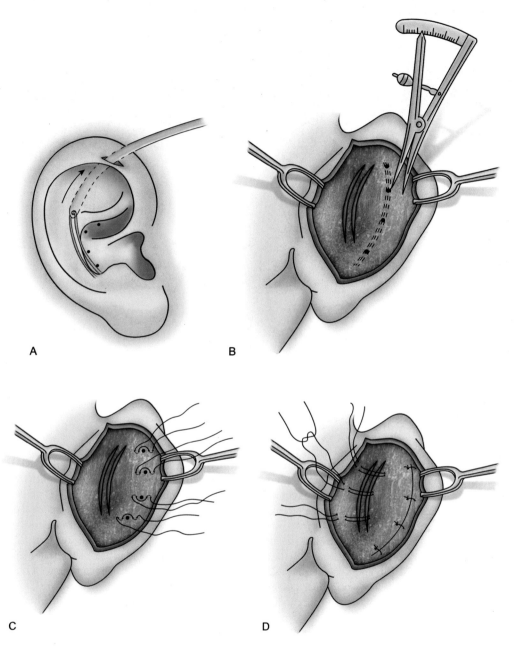

Figure 13-6. The method of Burstein. (A) Scaphal incision and anterior cartilage scoring with otobrader along proposed antihelical fold. (B) Posterior conchal cartilage trough incisions to weaken cartilage; location for placement of antihelical sutures is measured within scapha using calipers. (C) Scaphaconchal sutures placed. (D) Conchamastoid sutures placed. *(Continued)*

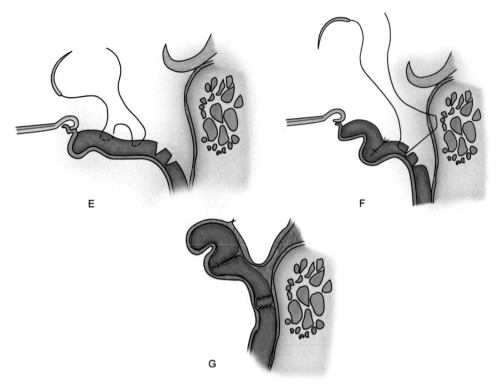

Figure 13-6. *(Continued)* (E) Axial view of full-thickness conchal cartilage incisions, posterior scaphal scoring, and antihelical suture placement. (F) Conchamastoid sutures placed. (G) Final auricular position.

helical rim. Unlike in Mustardé's description, these sutures are tightened down tightly rather than adjusted individually, as this makes interaural symmetry easier to achieve because it is easier to reproduce from side to side.

Conchal hypertrophy is addressed subsequently. The previously marked line designating the lateral conchal margin is used to indicate the proposed conchal scoring incisions. Two scoring incisions are made, paralleling the long axis of the ear. The first incision is made at the lateral limit of the concha. The second incision is made approximately 6 mm medial to the first one. This method is similar to the scaphal incisions described by Tanzer[20] for creation of the antihelical fold. The perichondrium is cut using microcautery and the cartilage is incised sharply with a scalpel through its full thickness, but preserving the anterior skin. Mattress sutures of 4-0 nylon are then placed between the distal edge of the most lateral incision and the mastoid periosteum. This corrects central ear prominence. If less conchal recession is desired, the sutures may be situated more medially on the concha. Burstein cautions against

bringing the most lateral point of the helix any closer than 18 mm from the scalp in order to prevent a stuck down appearance. Redundant skin is trimmed conservatively in an hourglass configuration at the conclusion of the case. In the case of an outstanding lobule, a soft tissue wedge is excised perpendicular to the long axis of the skin incision. The wound is then closed with a running 4-0 chromic gut suture.

In his review of 100 patients treated bilaterally over 10 years, Burstein reported consistently satisfying results with few complications. There were no infections and one postauricular hematoma was uneventfully evacuated in the office. Four ears suffered from mild relapse at the superior pole that was corrected, interestingly enough, simply by postauricular skin excision under local anesthesia. Four more ears required more aggressive treatment of recurrent protrusion by replacement of one or more mattress sutures. All eight recurrences were the result of suture failure or suture pull-through. These all occurred early in the postoperative course and were attributed to superficial suture placement and to inadequate cartilage scoring. Hypertrophic scars developed in three patients, all responding to medical management with topical and/or injectable steroids. The recurrence rate of 8% is similar to that reported elsewhere. This combined technique has proved for Burstein to be a powerful tool for the complete correction of all elements of the prominent ear.

Other Notable Combination Techniques

A novel approach to otoplasty was described by Burres[21] that he termed the anterior-posterior otoplasty **(Figure 13-7)**. This is a combined technique that allows graded control of helical and conchal

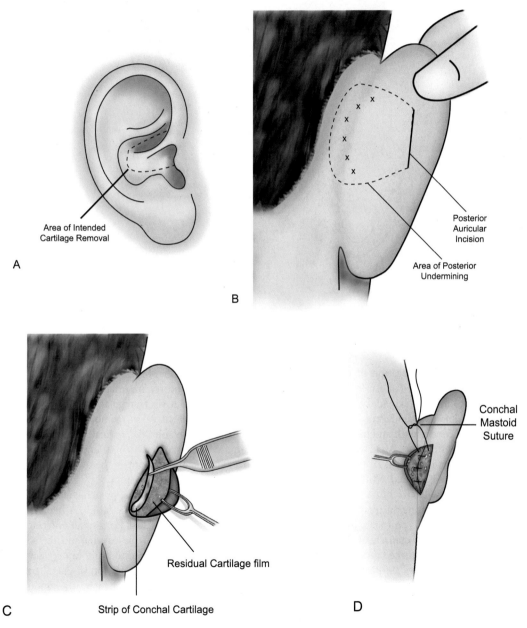

Figure 13-7. The method of Burres. (A) Semilunar area of conchal cartilage excision marked. (B) Small access posterior incision with limited undermining; X's indicate points of potential cartilage fixation. (C) Removal of conchal cartilage strip. (D) Conchamastoid suture placement. *(Continued)*

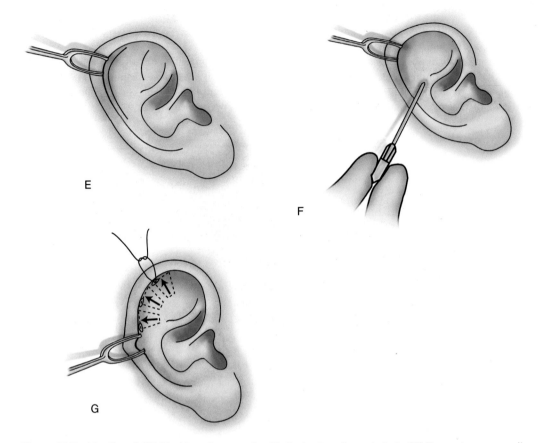

Figure 13-7. *(Continued)* (E) Marking of proposed antihelical suture line anteriorly. (F) Transcutaneous needle cartilage scoring. (G) Antihelical mattress suture placement.

angulation by the application of mattress sutures across areas of weakened or excised cartilage. A limited posterior incision is made overlying the posterior concha and skin undermining is restricted to the posterior concha itself and to the area overlying the mastoid periosteum. A curvilinear strip of lateral conchal cartilage about 20 to 30 mm long and 5 to 6 mm wide is excised. Mattress sutures of 4-0 Vicryl are then used to fix the concha to the mastoid, routinely overcorrecting the medial deflection by 5° to 10°. Medialization is promoted by excision of 5 or 6 mm of redundant postauricular skin.

Attention is then turned anteriorly where antihelical mattress sutures are placed percutaneously. The intended mattress suture lines are drawn in with gentian violet. Through several small access incisions on the anterior scapha, the central portion of the antihelix is scored longitudinally with a bent hypodermic needle. Mattress sutures of 4-0 nylon are then passed anteriorly via several stab incisions

made in the gutter of the scapha parallel to the helical rim. The sutures are oriented radially from the center of the fossa triangularis. They are passed through the cartilage on the horizontal passes and subcutaneously on the vertical passes. The skin around each stab incision is undermined with a needle allowing the knots to be oversewn with 6-0 chromic fast-absorbing sutures.

An anterior-posterior approach is also advocated by de la Fuente and Santamaría[22]. A hypertrophic concha is addressed first via a small anterior incision at the border of the concha and the scapha. This incision is designed to avoid unnecessary undermining. A semilunar portion of lateral conchal cartilage is excised as dictated by the amount of cartilage overlap when the ear is pushed posteriorly. Skin is not resected to avoid tension on the closure. This maneuver is followed by rasping of the intended antihelical cartilage through a small anterior incision until the cartilage is weak enough to turn back on its own. Deep conchamastoid sutures are placed only to reinforce the previous correction and are not intended to shape the ear. This is done via a narrow 3 to 5 mm elliptical posterior skin excision situated just above the sulcus. Rather than undermine widely, two to three subcutaneous posterior tunnels are dissected to permit suture placement. All incisions are closed with absorbable suture. The neo-antihelical roll may be splinted by placement of several 4-0 gut mattress sutures over adaptic rolls. This maintains the antihelical position for several days. When scaphal reduction is necessary, it is treated in much the same way as the conchal resection, with an incision located at the junction of the scapha and helix. Simple cuneiform excision may take care of an outstanding lobule. The authors believe that the ideal otoplasty method should use minimal incisions, dissection be limited to the defect, and should not cause foreign bodies such as permanent sutures to be retained in the ear. They have not reported problems with scarring of the anterior incisions.

Erol[23] has presented a true combination technique in 55 patients that is undertaken through a strictly anterior approach. This approach is designed so that the neurovascular structures of the ear are not disturbed on its posterior surface. All modern otoplasty maneuvers may be undertaken as necessary, including conchal reduction and setback, scaphal cartilage scoring, placement of buried mattress sutures, and aggressive retropositioning of the tail and superior pole. Few late complications were noted, comprising suture reaction in 1.8%, hidden helix in 3.6% and partial relapse in 3.6% that was readily treated with a single Kaye-type buried suture.

Epstein and colleagues[24] prefer a posterior approach with weakening of the posterior cartilage surface using an electrocautery knife (**Figure 13-8**). The intended antihelical reference points are marked anteriorly and posteriorly with the needle pull-through method described previously in this chapter. A posterior hourglass-shaped elliptical skin excision is designed completely on the posterior surface of the auricle. Wide undermining is followed by conchamastoid suture placement and conchal excision, if indicated, along the free edge at the external auditory meatus.

A spatula-tip cautery blade is used on cutting mode to create a smooth, partial thickness trough or gutter in the posterior scaphal cartilage along the previously marked line through the antihelix and both superior and inferior crura in a Y-shape. Extending

the troughs halfway to two-thirds of the way through the cartilage will usually facilitate folding without creating a sharp edge. Finally, scaphaconchal sutures of 4-0 clear nylon or Mersilene are placed and sequentially adjusted and tied down. Postoperative antibiotics are prescribed. This technique was applied in more than 60 patients with reliable results. No major complications were encountered including chondritis or skin abnormalities attributable to thermal injury. Revision procedures were performed in six ears for partial loss of correction.

Another large series publication of a combination technique was presented by Yugueros and Friedland[25]. In their favored method, three classic techniques are combined to treat the prominent ear. They make use of subcutaneous anterior scoring, antihelical mattress suturing, and conchamastoid setback with sutures. Postoperative analysis of long-term results in 100 consecutive patients revealed complication rates that were lower than in previously reported similar series, along with a high satisfaction rate.

Combination techniques have been very effective for many others. A combination cartilage cutting-molding method is the otoplasty procedure of choice for Ducic and Hilger[26]. Hell et al.,[27] used an approach in 312 patients that combined a dorsal skin excision, cartilage incision at the scaphaconchal border, anterior scoring of the superior crus, and conchal excision with cauda helicis resection as needed. Similarly, Gomulinski et al.,[28] prefer a method that mingles resection of the helical tail with single suture fixation, scoring of the scapha through an anterior approach, and redundant posterior soft tissues to set back the concha.

Numerous adjustments to cartilage-sparing techniques have been combined to preserve greater contour stability. Lazaridis et al.,[29] have modified a conventional scoring technique to better control cartilage folding. For this purpose, they combine three adjustable transfixion sutures with shallower scoring incisions. Their preferred suture material is 4-0 Vicryl since permanent sutures are not required to maintain the new contour. A closed anterior scoring technique fortified by suturing of the cartilage has also been advocated by Thomas and Fatah[30]. They prefer a buried Prolene suture, however. In 32 patients, one ear relapsed at the superior pole and another experienced a suture extrusion. Pilz et al.,[31] performed a modified scoring otoplasty in more than 300 patients with exemplary operative outcomes. Their technique utilizes a spherical

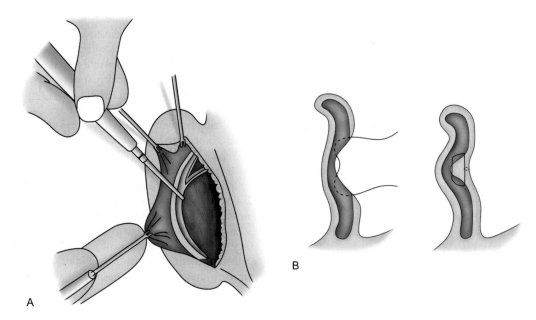

Figure 13-8. The method of Epstein. (A) Partial-thickness troughs created in posterior scaphal cartilage along desired antihelical and crural line with electrocautery spatula-tip blade. (B) Cross-sectional view demonstrating partial-thickness incision of cartilage with posterior mattress sutures.

metal head dermabrader to create postauricular furrowing followed by vertical mattress sutures. A modified scoring-suturing technique is also favored by Salgarello et al.,[32] whose particular procedure involves posterior access without skin excision, anterior scoring, and mattress sutures. There were few complications and aesthetic results were graded as good or very good in 95% of 135 patients recently studied. Benedict and Pirwitz[33] reported on their experience with a modified Kaye[34] otoplasty using minimal access in 442 ears. Key aspects of this technique combine permanent buried sutures with conservative cartilage-breaking methods through small incisions without extensive skin excision. Complications included residual or recurrent protrusion in 9.9%, suture reactions in 9.3%, early infections in 0.7%, prolonged sensitivity in 0.7%, and a single hypertrophic scar. According to the authors, a very strong cartilage framework and a very high conchal wall present limitations for this method and may account for the reasonably high incidence of reprotrusion noted in this review.

In the current section of this text, we have featured unique adaptations of every major known otoplasty technique along with nearly every combination and permutation thereof. While most every author reports highly satisfying outcomes with their specific method, in the next chapter, we will try to draw more standardized comparisons so that the reader may more comfortably cull techniques that are fitting to their practices.

References

1. Mustardé JC. The correction of prominent ears using simple mattress sutures. *Br J Plast Surg* 16:170, 1963.
2. Stënstrom SJ. A natural technique for correction of congenital ear deformities. *Br J Plast Surg* 99:562, 1963.
3. Converse JM, Nigro A, Wilson FA, Johnson N. A technique for surgical correction of lop ears. *Plast Reconstr Surg* 15:411, 1955.
4. Horlock N, Misra A, Gault DT. The postauricular fascial flap as an adjunct to Mustardé and Furnas-type otoplasty. *Plast Reconstr Surg* 108(6):1487–90, 2001.
5. Stucker FJ, Christiansen TA. The lateral conchal resection otoplasty. *Laryngoscope* 87:58–62, 1977.
6. Stucker FJ, Vora NM, Lian TS. Otoplasty: an analysis of technique over a 33-year period. *Laryngoscope* 113:952–6, 2003.
7. Burningham AR, Stucker FJ. Otoplasty technique: How I do it. *Facial Plast Surg Clin N Am* 14:73–77, 2006.
8. Farrior RT. A method of otoplasty. *Arch Otolaryngol* 69:26–34, 1959.

9. Farrior RT. Otoplasty: surgery for protruding ears. In: Otolaryngology. Vol. 3. Hagerstown, MD: *Harper and Row Publishers, Inc.;* 1974: 1–23.

10. Scharer SA, Farrior EH, Farrior RT. Retrospective analysis of the Farrior technique for otoplasty. *Arch Facial Plast Surg* 9:167–73, 2007.

11. Stal S, Spira M. Long-term results in otoplasty. *Facial Plast Surg* 2:153–65, 1985.

12. Messner AH, Crysdale WS. Otoplasty: clinical protocol and long-term results. *Arch Otolaryngol Head Neck Surg* 122:773–7, 1996.

13. Caouette-Laberge L, Guay N, Bortoluzzi P, Belleville C. Otoplasty: anterior scoring technique and results in 500 cases. *Plast Reconstr Surg* 105(2):504–15., 2000.

14. Crikelair GF, Cosman B. Another solution for the problem of the prominent ear. *Ann Surg* 160:314, 1964.

15. Sénéchal B, Chauffeté JP, Sénéchal G. Complications et échecs des otoplasties. *Ann Otolaryngol Chir Cervicofac* 100:493, 1983.

16. Elliott RA Jr. Complications in the treatment of prominent ears. *Clin Plast Surg* 17:305, 1990.

17. Spira M. Otoplasty: what I do now- a 30-year perspective. *Plast Reconstr Surg* 104(3):834–40, 1999.

18. Cohen SR, Burstein FD. Protruding ear. In: Spitz L, Coran AG, eds. Rob and Smith's Operative Surgery. *London: Chapman and Hall Medical*, pp. 76–85, 1995.

19. Burstein FD. Cartilage-sparing complete otoplasty technique: a 10-year experience in 100 patients. *J Craniofacial Surg* 14(4):521–5, 2003.

20. Tanzer RC. The correction of prominent ears. *Plast Reconstr Surg* 23:1, 1962.

21. Burres S. The anterior-posterior otoplasty. *Arch Otolaryngol Head Neck Surg* 124:181–5, 1998.

22. de la Fuente A, Santamaría AB. Minimally invasive otoplasty. *Eur J Plast Surg* 21:249–53, 1998.

23. Erol OO. New modification in otoplasty: anterior approach. *Plast Reconstr Surg* 107(1):193–202., 2001.

24. Epstein JS, Kabaker SS, Swerdloff J. The "Electric" otoplasty. *Arch Facial Plast Surg* 1:204–7, 1999.

25. Yugueros P, Friedland JA. Otoplasty: the experience of 100 consecutive patients. *Plast Reconstr Surg* 108(4):1045–51, 2001.

26. Ducic Y, Hilger PA. Effective step-by-step technique for the surgical treatment of protruding ears. *J Otolaryngol* 28(2):59–64, 1999.

27. Hell B, Garbea D, Heissler E, Klein M, Gath H, Langford A. Otoplasty: a combined approach to different structures of the auricle. *Int J Oral Maxillofac Surg* 26(6):408–13, 1997.

28. Gomulinski L, Mauduy M, Saterre J. Our experience of otoplasty based on the study of the cartilaginous frame, especially the tail of the helix. *Ann Chir Plast Esthet* 50(3):206–15, 2005.

29. Lazaridis N, Tilaveridis I, Dimitrakopoulos I, Karakasis D. Correction of the protruding ear with a modified anterior scoring technique. *J Oral Maxillofac Surg* 56(3):307–13, 1998.

30. Thomas SS, Fatah F. Closed anterior scoring for prominent-ear correction revisited. *Br J Plast Surg* 54(7):581–7, 2001.

31. Pilz S, Hintringer T, Bauer M. Otoplasty using a spherical metal head dermabrador to form a retroauricular furrow: five-year results. *Aesthetic Plast Surg* 19(1):83–91, 1995.

32. Salgarello M, Gasperoni C, Montagnese A, Farallo E. Otoplasty for prominent ears: a versatile combined technique to master the shape of the ear. *Otolaryngol Head Neck Surg* 137(2):224–7, 2007.

33. Benedict M, Pirwitz KU. Minimally invasive otoplasty. *HNO* 53(3):230–7, 2005.

34. Kaye BL. A simplified method for correcting the prominent ear. *Plast Reconst Surg* 52:184, 1967.

14

Comparison of Otoplasty Techniques

Peter A. Adamson, MD, FRCSC, FACS and
Jason A. Litner, MD, FRCSC

Introduction

The plastic surgical literature is often impugned for its highly subjective makeup and for the poor quality of its evidence to support accepted practices. Indeed, a casual perusal of most pertinent journals reveals a plethora of articles that highlight personal experiences in the fashion of "How I do it" commentaries with a notable deficiency of basic science content. While interesting, these editorials do not permit very valuable comparisons to be made between techniques. Surgeons have been less inclined to embark upon the arduous task of quantifying their postoperative results. Governments and private insurers, on the other hand, are demanding more of medical practitioners in the way of evidence-based practices to support payment for services. Since elective cosmetic procedures are not influenced by such forces, they have not yet been rigorously subjected to high-quality comparative clinical testing.

Randomized, blinded trials occupy the highest tier of clinical assessment in terms of quality of evidence. Otoplasty, as with other plastic surgical techniques, does not lend itself well to randomized, controlled comparisons because of its elective nature. There are no such articles in the otoplasty literature. A slightly less worthy evaluation involves direct comparison of techniques in a nonrandomized and noncontrolled manner. In this tier, many factors are not controlled for and bias is not completely eliminated; however, the studies utilize objective, quantitative comparators so that proper inferences can be made. There is a handful of this type of assessment in the otoplasty literature. Finally, noncomparative, nonstandardized evaluations that rely on qualitative parameters to draw their conclusions occupy the lowest tier of evidential quality. Most articles in the otoplasty literature will fall into this category.

Objective measurements are uncommonly used in otoplasty papers. Rather, subjective outcome measures are often employed in their stead. In point of fact, reasonable objective measures do exist for the assessment of plastic surgery results[1]. Apart from cephalometric angles and measures, specific independent goals of otoplastic surgery have been described in detail by McDowell[2] and Wright[3]. In this chapter, we will highlight existing comparisons of otoplastic techniques in both the human and animal literature in an effort to extract some meaning for the clinical practice of otoplastic surgery.

Surgical Technique

Direct Comparisons of Otoplasty Techniques

The Edinburgh Experience

Mandal and colleagues[4] reported the Edinburgh experience of various otoplasty methods in 203 patients over a 5-year span. In this study, they attempted to compare the outcomes of three techniques: the anterior cartilage-scoring method (Group A), the posterior cartilage-suturing method (Group B), and the posterior cartilage-suturing method with advancement of a postauricular fascial flap (Group C) as proposed by Horlock[5]. The authors retrospectively reviewed their single-institution experience with these three techniques. Exclusion criteria were unilateral otoplasty; primary surgery done elsewhere; associated deformities other than prominent ears; and operations involving a combination of methods. Group A contained 68 patients, Group B had 94 patients, and Group C consisted of 41 patients. Between-group demographic data were comparable. Primary outcome measures were early and late postoperative complications, recurrence rates, reoperation rates, and patient and doctor satisfaction. Finally, patient photographs were assessed on a visual analog scale by a blinded lay observer and by a blinded physician to evaluate overall appearance and symmetry. All procedures were performed by either a consultant or specialist registrar.

Patients in Group A had their otoplasties performed using the classic Chongchet method[6]. In Group B, a combination of the classic Mustardé[7] and Furnas[8] suture techniques was used, employing a variety of suture materials including 4-0 nylon, 4-0 clear Prolene, and 4-0 PDS. In Group C, this same technique was combined with a posterior fascial flap for internal suture coverage as described by Horlock and Gault[5]. The flap was replaced over the posterior cartilage after suture placement and fixed to the inside of the anterior leading skin margin with 5-0 Vicryl rapide. Operating time in this group took longer than in Groups A and B.

Overall, comparison of operative results favored Group C. However, a key weakness of this study is the lack of statistical analysis of the data. Early complications such as bleeding and delayed healing were greatest in Group B and least in Group C. Likewise, late complications were fewest in Group C. Though complications were reasonably few in general, Group A experienced the highest rate of anterior skin necrosis, residual pain, and cartilage notching or irregularities. In contrast, suture granuloma, suture extrusion, and prominent scarring featured more prominently in Group B. Recurrence rates in Groups A, B, and C were 11%, 8%, and 4.8%, respectively. Re-operation rates for recurrence were 8.8%, 6%, and 3.6% in the same order. The ratings of aesthetic outcomes by both the lay observer and physician also favored Group C.

The authors concluded that the cartilage-scoring method, in their unit, resulted in unacceptably high rates of serious complications such as skin necrosis and cartilage destruction. Although these rates were comparable with those of other reports, the cartilage-suturing technique emerged as a safer procedure in their estimation. Avoidance of anterior dissection substantially curtailed the risk of hematoma and skin necrosis. In this study, suture techniques also resulted in fewer recurrences and revision surgeries, although suture extrusions did occur at a rate of roughly 3% in the suture-only group. The incidence of suture extrusion fell to 1% in Group C when the posterior fascial flap was performed.

The Feldkirch/Zürich Experience

In 2003, Kompatscher and colleagues[9] published their direct comparison of two popular otoplasty methods, the Francesconi otoplasty[10] and the Converse otoplasty[11]. The Francesconi otoplasty comprises a blending of the anterior subperichondrial scoring method of Stenström[12] and the dorsal buried mattress suture technique of Mustardé[7]. Francesconi incorporated anterior scoring into his technique because he found that the mattress suture technique, used alone, often resulted in a certain degree of re-protrusion. In addition, it could not adequately address the issue of conchal hyperplasia.

Prior to this direct study, Kompatscher and colleagues had begun to increasingly favor the Francesconi method because their impression of the Converse otoplasty was that it resulted in too many 'unnatural ears' in their clinic. This quality control study was undertaken during an 11-year period in which both methods were being used routinely. From a cohort of 281 patients operated on during that time, a sample of 28 primary otoplasty patients was randomly chosen. Group 1 comprised 14 Francesconi otoplasty patients and Group 2 consisted of 14 Converse otoplasty patients. The groups were matched for demographic variables. All patients had conchal hyperplasia, either alone or in addition to an unfurled antihelix. The study protocol called for exclusion of patients with other ear anomalies, those having unilateral otoplasty, and those with a follow-up period of less than 6 months. Major outcome measures were derived from retrospective review of patient records, digital photos, and personal examination by an independent plastic surgeon. Objective parameters included the physiognomic length and width of the ear; the superior, medial, and inferior cephaloauricular distances; and the conchoscaphal angle. The incidence of complications was gleaned from a review of the medical record. Judgments of symmetry, contour, and overall satisfaction were made on a visual analog scale by both the patient and the independent plastic surgeon.

Results indicated that the anatomic parameters were similar between groups except for medial and inferior cephaloauricular distances, which were lesser in the Francesconi group. In both groups, these measures were slightly less than for a 'normal' reference population[13], indicating a slight overcorrection. A tendency towards some overcorrection has been confirmed by other retrospective reviews[14]. This is just as well, since patients often wish for a slight overcorrection, and do not find undercorrection nearly as acceptable. The conchoscaphal angle was 90° or less in all Group 1 patients, but more than 90° in 57% of the Converse group. These findings were statistically significant.

Only one early complication occurred, in the Converse group (a hematoma), and this was evacuated conservatively. Unsatisfactory results were rated according to very strict criteria[15]. According to this very rigid Strasser evaluation system, imperfections were noted to be quite common in both groups, although much more so in the Converse Group. Statistically significant differences were noted favoring the Francesconi Group in judgments of asymmetry and undercorrection, while a statistical trend favored the same group for measures of abnormal ear lobe protrusion and upper pole protrusion. Finally, the examiner's satisfaction rating was significantly better for the Francesconi method. The patients' own ratings trended towards statistical significance in favor of the Francesconi method as well, although both groups were very approving of their results.

Although representative sample sizes were small in this study, the authors concluded that the Francesconi method led to a higher rate of correction of protrusion, both objectively and subjectively, and to higher surgeon satisfaction rates.

The Bologna Experience

Panettiere et al.,[16] reported on their experience on 63 consecutive patients operated on over an 11-year period. During the first 5 years, 33 patients (Group A) were treated using a resection technique for their antihelical defects. In the last 6 years, 30 patients (Group B) underwent cartilage weakening and suture otoplasty for similar defects. The degree of severity of the deformities was judged to be comparable between the two groups by an independent plastic surgeon. The groups were similar in age, sex, and laterality.

Posterior approaches were undertaken in both groups. In Group A, the cartilage was transected along the desired line of the antihelix starting about 2 cm above the anterior insertion site of the helix and following a smooth arc to the lateral conchal margin. The cartilage edges were then oversewn with nonabsorbable full-thickness mattress sutures of 5-0 Prolene alternating with 5-0 PDS. The muscular-perichondrial layer was coapted separately with 5-0 PDS. In Group B, cartilage weakening was carried out by longitudinal scoring of the posterior aspect of the antihelix using either fine rasps or a blade, following the description of Maniglia[17]. The line of scoring was identical to the line of transection noted above. Cartilage-sutures and muscular-perichondrial sutures were performed as described above. Conchal hypertrophy, if present, was treated in both groups by segmental resection and suturing of the apposed edges followed by placement of conchamastoid sutures. All other parameters were maintained consistently between the two groups such that treatment of the antihelix was the only real difference.

Primary outcome measures were the incidence of complications and the assessment by an independent blinded plastic surgeon of the suitability of correction and the overall aesthetic result. No major complications occurred in either group. Residual protrusion was noted in 4% of patients in Group A as compared to 2% in Group B. The overall aesthetic result was judged to be similar in both groups. Nevertheless, an excessively sharp antihelical fold was observed in nearly all Group A patients (92%) whereas this phenomenon was not seen in Group B. Scoring of the cartilage with the rasp was noted to be quicker, easier, more reproducible, and safer than was scoring with a knife. There was a lower risk of inadvertent full thickness incisions with this form of scoring. No significant difference was found between the two groups in the degree of patient satisfaction. The authors concluded that a cartilage rasping and suturing method has provided them the best aesthetic contour without sacrificing long-term effectiveness and stability.

The Experience of Others

Härtel and Bonitz[14], in the German-language literature, compared their experiences with the Haecker and Joseph otoplasty in 77 patients to their use of the Converse method in 70 patients. In a retrospective, subjectively judged review, they found an unsatisfactory outcome in 12.9% of Converse procedures compared to just 2.6% of Haecker and Joseph procedures.

Goode et al.,[18] compared the incidence of postoperative loss of correction with reprotrusion in a mattress suture otoplasty technique versus a cartilage -cutting technique. In their study, recurrence was greater with the cartilage-cutting otoplasty (13.6% of 44 patients) than when a cartilage-sparing method was used (4.8% of 126 patients).

Tan[19] undertook a retrospective study of 119 patients under the age of 16 who had undergone otoplasty by one of two methods during a four-year period. Patients were treated using either the Mustardé technique (45 patients) or an anterior scoring method (101 patients). Overall, patient acceptance of the results was obtained from a questionnaire and the case sheets were reviewed. Although there was no difference in the final acceptance of both methods, a significantly larger number of cases treated with the Mustardé technique needed reoperation. This occurrence was blamed on the use of white silk suture material that, according to the author, was the inciting cause of frequent stitch complications.

Literature Reviews of Otoplasty Techniques

The otoplasty literature is replete with reviews of long-term series belonging to individual surgeons or single institutions. Yet, to our knowledge, few studies have attempted to analyze and categorize these results in a uniform way. In 2005, Richards et al.[20] accomplished just that. They reviewed all articles on the topic published in the English language literature between 1977 and 2002. Inclusion criteria were postoperative follow-up for a minimum of 6 months; consistent surgical technique applied to all cases; primary surgery only; and analysis of postoperative results available with consistent quantifiable criteria. Results were considered to be objective if they were reported according to anatomical measures or to accepted criteria[2,3]. Subjective assessments were reclassified as being satisfactory or unsatisfactory so that inter-study comparisons could be made.

Of the 149 papers identified by the search, only 12 met all criteria for inclusion, illustrating the fact that most articles on the subject are purely descriptive in nature. Four fundamentally distinct techniques were identified among the included studies. These comprised suturing alone, scoring alone, scoring and suturing, and cartilage-cutting

techniques. Only five of these papers used one of the objective grading systems mentioned above.

The percentage of patients who were dissatisfied with their results was low in all groups. This was the case in 7.1% of suture only patients, 4.8% of rasping only cases, 4% of those undergoing rasping and suturing, and 5.2% of cartilage-cutting cases. These differences were not statistically significant. Overall dissatisfaction in all cases was 4.3% for patients and 7.7% for surgeons. This difference was not statistically significant, although sample sizes were small. The greatest incidence of complications was noted in suture techniques. Suture extrusion occurred in 12.5%, mostly involving late extrusion of Mersilene sutures. These occurred, on average, 12 to 24 months postoperatively and did not alter auricular contour after removal. Other complications including pain, bleeding, infection, and keloid formation occurred in less than 5% of patients regardless of the otoplasty method used. Evaluation of quantitative criteria proved problematic in this study because measures were sufficiently disparate so as to render them incomparable. The authors concluded that, based on this review, all surgical techniques appear equally successful when qualitative factors are evaluated.

Additional reviews simply give an account of complication rates without making an attempt to standardize these results for comparative purposes. These will be highlighted in the next section dedicated to otoplasty complications and aesthetic pitfalls.

Animal Comparisons of Otoplasty Techniques

A number of animal studies have assessed the effects of various otoplasty techniques on cartilage deformation. The New Zealand white rabbit model appears to be the accepted standard for such appraisals. Rohrich et al.,[21] studied a multitude of techniques in 42 rabbit ears including anterior or posterior scoring, horizontal or vertical mattress sutures, and scoring-suturing combinations. After 8 weeks, suture methods alone or in combination with scoring of the cartilage were able to maintain an angulation significantly closer to the desired 90° than did scoring used alone. The greatest efficacy was observed with horizontal mattress sutures. This reflection was confirmed on histologic analysis, wherein suture methods demonstrated a significant increase in cartilage hyperplasia compared to other techniques that showed only mild to moderate histologic changes. These findings support the use of mattress sutures to remodel auricular cartilage.

Weinzweig et al.,[22] studied the effects of three different otoplasty methods in New Zealand white rabbits. Eighteen rabbits were divided into three equal groups. A subcutaneous pocket was developed on the posterior surface of each animal's ears. In all animals, the perichondrium of one ear was stripped while that of the other ear was preserved. Otoplasties were performed, as in other comparative studies, using either the method of Converse, Mustardé, or Stenström. Permanent sutures were inserted in all groups to help maintain the correction. These sutures were cut at varying intervals of 1, 2, 4, and 6 weeks. Necropsy was undertaken 1 week after sutures were cut. On histomorphologic analysis, the antihelical fold best maintained its shape in the group in which the anterior perichondrium was rasped. Stabilization of the newly formed fold was reinforced in this group by formation of a fibrocartilaginous cap over the rasped surface. Significantly less anterior cartilage proliferation was discovered in the other two groups. A fibrous cap was not observed in these samples. Stripping of the perichondrium stimulated cartilaginous proliferation in all groups. The ears in which the sutures were cut at 1 week experienced a loss of correction while an increasing cartilaginous proliferation noted subsequent to one week was seen to stabilize the correction.

In 1984, DeMars and colleagues[23] examined the durability of various otoplasty techniques in the rabbit model. The techniques studied were suture placement with or without concomitant cartilage scoring and isolated cartilage abrasion. In ten rabbits, the ear was abraded along its posterior surface and folded forward to attain a 90° angle, and the correction was reinforced with nylon sutures. The same procedure was performed on the opposite ear, omitting the cartilage abrasion. In four more rabbits, abrasion was undertaken by itself without suture support. Finally, in one rabbit, undermining of the posterior skin was completed on its own in both ears. In contrast to the findings of Weinzweig[22] noted earlier, ears reshaped with suture alone best maintained the original angle while those treated with suture and abrasion did not maintain the desired conformation.

More recently, Hagerty et al.,[24] compared the histologic changes and durability associated with rabbit ear folding using one of three techniques. Twenty-six ears in thirteen New Zealand white rabbits were divided into three treatment groups: bent cartilage (9 ears), cut cartilage (9 ears), and endoscopic

cartilage abrasion (8 ears). All ears were folded transversely over 180 degrees and were maintained with external mattress sutures. Sutures were removed at 1 to 6 weeks postoperatively and the ears were followed for a further 4 weeks. At final measure, mean ear angles were 13 degrees in the bent ear (control) group, 84 degrees in the cut cartilage group, and 132 degrees in the abraded cartilage group. Perichondrial thickening was noted on the convex surface upon histologic sectioning of all ears. Fibrocartilage was produced in both the cut and abraded cartilage groups, although it appeared more fibrous in the cut cartilage group.

It would appear, overall, that animal studies have produced mixed findings in support of either cartilage scoring or cartilage suturing techniques. It is abundantly clear, however, from the few direct comparative studies presented, that cartilage-sparing methods have proven more effective than their cartilage-cutting counterparts in obtaining and maintaining correction of the protruding ear with a more favorable aesthetic contour, and with a low incidence of complications. In the next section, we will analyze the most frequently encountered complications and aesthetic pitfalls associated with otoplasty, their causes and management, and, most importantly, how these may be judiciously avoided.

References

1. Wood SH, Tarar MN. Outcome audit in plastic surgery: the Cambridge classification. *Br J Plast Surg* 47:122, 1994.
2. McDowell AJ. Goals in otoplasty for protruding ears. *Plast Reconstr Surg* 41:17–27, 1968.
3. Wright WK. Otoplasty goals and principles. *Arch Otolaryngol* 92:568–72, 1970.
4. Mandal A, Bahia H, Ahmad T, Stewart KJ. Comparison of cartilage scoring and cartilage sparing otoplasty – a study of 203 cases. *J Plast Reconstr Aesthetic Surg* 59:1170–76, 2006.
5. Horlock N, Misra A, Gault DT. The postauricular fascial flap as an adjunct to Mustardé and Furnas-type otoplasty. *Plast Reconstr Surg* 108(6):1487–90, 2001.
6. Chongchet V. A method for antihelix reconstruction. *Br J Plast Surg* 16:268, 1963.
7. Mustardé JC. The correction of prominent ears using simple mattress sutures. *Br J Plast Surg* 16:170, 1963.
8. Furnas DW. Correction of prominent ears by conchamastoid sutures. *Plast Reconstr Surg* 42:189, 1968.
9. Kompatscher P, Schuler CH, Clemens S, Seifert B, Beer GM. The cartilage-sparing versus the cartilage-cutting technique: a retrospective quality control

comparison of the Francesconi and Converse otoplasties. *Aesthetic Plast Surg* 27(6):446–53, 2003.

10. Francesconi G, Grassi C, Chiocchetti FC. La nostra esperienza nel trattamento chirugico dell' orecchio ad ansa. *Acta Otorhinol Ital* 2:163–82, 1982.

11. Converse JM, Nigro A, Wilson FA, Johnson N. A technique for surgical correction of lop ears. *Plast Reconstr Surg* 15:411, 1955.

12. Stenström SJ. A "natural" technique for correction of congenital prominent ears. *Plast Reconstr Surg* 32:509, 1963.

13. Wodak E. Über die stellung und form der menschlichen ohrmuschel. *Arch Klin Exp Ohren-Nasen-Kehlkopfheilk* 188:381–6, 1967.

14. Härtel J, Bonitz R. Spätergebnisse von Korrekturoperationen abstehender ohrmuscheln. *Zent bl Chir* 115:161–4, 1990.

15. Strasser E. Application of an objective grading system for the evaluation of cosmetic surgical results. *Plast Reconstr Surg* 109:1733–40, 2002.

16. Panettiere P, Marchetti L, Accorsi D, Del Gaudio GA. Otoplasty: a comparison of techniques for antihelical defects treatment. *Aesth Plast Surg* 27:462–5, 2004.

17. Maniglia AJ, Maniglia JJ, Witten BR. Otoplasty: an eclectic technique. *Laryngoscope* 87:1359–68, 1977.

18. Goode RL, Proffitt SD, Rafaty FM. Complications of otoplasty. *Arch Otolaryngol* 91(4):352–5, 1970.

19. Tan KH. Long-term survey of prominent ear surgery: a comparison of two methods. *Br J Plast Surg* 39(2):270–3, 1986.

20. Richards SD, Jebreel A, Capper R. Otoplasty: a review of the surgical techniques. *Clin Otolaryngol* 30:2–8, 2005.

21. Rohrich RJ, Friedman RM, Liland DL. Comparison of otoplasty techniques in the rabbit model. *Ann Plast Surg* 34(1):43–7, 1995.

22. Weinzweig N, Chen L, Sullivan WG. Histomorphology of neochondrogenesis after antihelical fold creation: a comparison of three otoplasty techniques in the rabbit. *Ann Plast Surg* 33(4):371–6, 1994.

23. DeMars RV, Schenden MJ, Manders EK, Graham WP 3rd. The permanence of otoplasty in the rabbit ear: a comparison of techniques. *Ann Plast Surg* 13(3):195–8, 1984.

24. Hagerty TA, Barone EJ, Cohen IK. Endoscopic otoplasty in the rabbit model: effect of mechanical abrasion on ear cartilage deformation. *Plast Reconstr Surg* 101(2):487–93, 1998.

15

COMPLICATIONS OF OTOPLASTY

PETER A. ADAMSON, MD, FRCSC, FACS AND
JASON A. LITNER, MD, FRCSC

Introduction

Cosmetic otoplasty is a satisfying operation for both patient and surgeon, and pleasing aesthetic outcomes are obtained in the great majority of cases. Major complications are decidedly uncommon after otoplasty although minor complications have been noted by some authors to occur with astonishing frequency regardless of otoplasty technique[1-4]. Jeffery[1] has reported a complication rate of 23.8% with an anterior scoring technique in a review of 122 cases; however, the reoperation rate for recurrence was only 3.3%. Tan[2] found an unacceptably high recurrence rate (24%) following a posterior suture method. This was attributed to the presence of sinus tracts and wound infection ascribed to the use of white silk sutures. Farrior's combination technique[3] was recently reviewed in 75 patients with an occurrence of minor complications in 39% of patients studied. The most frequently seen problems in their review were suture reaction or extrusion in 21% of cases and reprotrusion in 22% of patients. Calder and Naasan[4] reviewed their experience of complications in 562 otoplasties performed by the anterior scoring method. The most frequent complications were asymmetry in 11% and recurrence in 8% followed by infection, keloid scarring, hemorrhage, and anterior skin necrosis.

The incidence of complications following otoplasty varies widely in the literature largely based on the degree of vigilance in recording these problems. Since most complications are minor and sometimes immaterial to the final aesthetic result, a heightened level of diligence is required if one is to provide a complete reporting of all such problems. Since most studies comprise retrospective chart reviews, less ominous complications may often be underreported in such series. Those studies that adhere to more rigorous objective standards of comparison such as those put forth by McDowell[5] and Wright[6] will almost invariably record a higher incidence of minor complications. This apparently higher complication rate may, in fact, reflect a reporting bias rather than a true difference in experience, a detail that will be kept in mind by the analytical reader.

Complications may be organized according to frequency, severity, and temporal association with the surgical procedure. It behooves the otoplastic surgeon to be well-versed in the most frequent and the most morbid complications related to otoplasty, and to communicate these effectively to prospective surgical candidates in the preoperative period. Patients who are enlightened to the potential problems that might affect the postoperative ear are generally tolerant of minor healing concerns and do not often seek revision surgery. Mandatory revision surgery has been estimated to encompass only about 2% percent of otoplasty cases[7]. This incidence compares favorably to other cosmetic facial procedures and underscores the general level of happiness associated with otoplasty outcomes.

A thorough review of otoplasty complications has recently been undertaken by the senior author[8]. It is important to distinguish unsatisfactory cosmetic results from true surgical complications and so, in an effort to separate the two, the issue of aesthetic shortfalls will be attended to in the final chapter of this volume. In this penultimate chapter, we will discuss real surgical complications, both frequent and sporadic, with an eye towards their prevention and management. A comparison of the incidence of significant complications associated with various techniques among large patient series is illustrated in **Table 15-1**. While this comparison is undermined somewhat by the lack of conformity of assessment criteria used in the literature, it is still revealing. In the following text, potential otoplasty complications are grouped as early or late complications and are presented in descending order of frequency.

Early Complications

Early complications occur within hours to days of the procedure and most often include the following:

Postoperative Nausea and Vomiting

The coincidence of postoperative nausea and vomiting (PONV) is relatively high after otoplasty, especially in the pediatric population. The incidence of PONV was found to be from 15 to 40% with the administration of antiemetic prophylaxis and as high as 52 to 85% without such prophylaxis[9]. The postulated mechanism for such a high association is surgical stimulation of a theoretical auriculoemetic reflex. Arnold's nerve or the auriculotemporal nerve has been suggested as the afferent limb of this postulated reflex arc[9,10]. The same authors found that pretreatment with transdermal scopolamine[9] or ondansetron[10] resulted in a significant decrease in PONV and in time to resumption of oral intake. Pretreatment should be administered on or before induction of anesthesia for maximum benefit.

General anesthesia may account for the higher incidence of PONV in the pediatric age group because adults may often tolerate local anesthesia for this procedure. At least one group of investigators has examined the use of local anesthesia with sedation for pediatric otoplasty[11]. They found that they could obtain comparable surgical results with less need for a prolonged hospital stay and substantially decreased PONV. There was zero incidence of PONV or admission to hospital in 41 children who received only local anesthesia compared to nearly half of 44 children administered general anesthesia who experienced vomiting, of which two were severe enough to warrant hospital admission. The incidence of PONV is neither trivial nor relevant only to patient comfort. A rise in blood pressure and capillary blood flow to the operated area as a result of PONV, may increase the very real risk of postoperative hematoma. Any finding that significantly decreases the incidence of causal factors for this complication is a most welcome addition to the body of knowledge on otoplasty.

Postoperative Pain

Mild pain and discomfort is a frequent result of otoplasty surgery, given the many sensory afferents that supply the external ear. Severe pain, on the other hand, especially if unilateral, is ominous and should raise the surgeon's suspicion of an impending hematoma, infection, or serious wound complication. Severe pain in the first 48 hours most frequently indicates a hematoma or a pressure-related injury to the auricle because of careless dressing application. Severe pain encountered in the ensuing 3 to 5 days should raise warnings of an early infection or impending tissue necrosis. In all such cases, a high index of suspicion is warranted and should provoke removal of the dressings, close inspection of the operative site, and prompt initiation of treatment.

Although postoperative pain does not play a prominent role in otoplasty, recent advances in perioperative pain management have led to improved postoperative comfort relating to decreased neuroendocrine stress. Ferraro et al.,[12] found perioperative use of remifentanil to be superior to combined propofol and midazolam in ensuring intraoperative and postoperative comfort. Supplemental use of local anesthesia in the operative field has also been shown to decrease postoperative narcotic requirements and to diminish pain scores, regardless of whether general anesthesia or monitored sedation was used[13]. There is no significant difference in postoperative pain regardless of whether regional nerve blockade or direct local infiltration is used, although the latter does aid in hemostasis[14]. Some authors[15] have suggested the choice of ropivacaine as a local anesthetic agent as a more desirable alternative to the more commonly used lidocaine or bupivacaine because of its more favorable risk profile.

Skin Reactions

Early skin reactions following otoplasty usually involve a contact allergic dermatitis or inflammatory

TABLE 15-1 Comparison of Otoplasty Complications by Technique, Author, Year, and Number of Patients

Technique	Method	Author	Year	No. of patients (ears)	Hematoma & Bleeding (%)	Infection (%)	Suture Reaction/ Extrusion (%)	Skin Ulceration/ Necrosis (%)	Hypertrophic/ Keloid Scarring (%)
Cartilage Cutting	Pitanguy Island flap ± conchal excision	Bartkowski et al.	2001	80	3.8	–	–	–	–
	Anterior skin + conchal excision, posterior mattress sutures	Bauer et al.	2002	47 (87)	0	0	0	0	0
	Cartilage tubing, anterior scoring	Peker and Celikoz	2002	178 (343)	7.9	0	0	0	1.7
	Posterior incision + mattress sutures	Panettiere et al.	2004	33	0	0	0	0	0
	Cartilage tubing ± conchal excision	Kompatscher et al.	2004	14	7	–	–	–	14
	Pitanguy Island flap + SC ± conchal excision	Werdin et al.	2007	278 (551)	1*	2*	–	–	0.7*
Cartilage Scoring	Incision + anterior scoring	Chongchet	1963	21	5	–	–	–	–
	Anterior scoring	Tan	1986	101	8	–	–	–	–
	Incision + anterior scoring	Calder and Naasan	1994	562	2	5.2	0	1.4	2.1
	Anterior scoring ± SC	Jeffery	1999	122	3.4	–	0	1.7	8*
	Anterior scoring + SC	Azuara	2000	(100)	–	–	–	–	–
	Anterior scoring ± conchal excision	Nordzell	2000	80 (160)	0	0	–	0	2.5
	Percutaneous anterior scoring + SC	Bulstrode et al.	2003	114 (214)	0.9	3.5	0	0	1.8
	Anterior scoring + SC	Nolst Trenité	2004	65	0	0	0	–	–
	Posterior scoring + mattress sutures	Panettiere et al.	2004	30	0	0	0	0	0
	Anterior abrasion ± CM	Di Mascio et al.	2004	40 (75)	7.5	–	–	–	–
	Anterior scoring	Raunig	2005	(302)	0*	0*	–	–	0*
	Anterior scoring	Mandal et al.	2006	68	1.5	1.5	–	0.7	1.4
	Anterior scoring + CM	Bhatti and Donavan	2007	34 (68)	2.9	2.9	0	0	0
Cartilage Suturing	SC + CM	Rigg	1979	101	–	–	11	–	–
	SC	Minderjahn et al.	1980	135	–	–	–	–	–
	SC	Attwood and Evans	1985	52	2.2	3.8	4.6	–	–
	SC	Tan	1986	45	33	–	15	–	–
	Modified SC	Koch et al.	1991	340	0	–	–	–	–
	Posterior SC +CM	Adamson et al.	1991	62 (119)	0.8*	0*	8.4*	0*	1.6*
	Posterior SC +CM	Vuyk et al.	1994	62 (117)	–	–	12.8*	–	–

TABLE 15-1 Comparison of Otoplasty Complications by Technique, Author, Year, and Number of Patients (Continued)

Technique	Method	Author	Year	No. of patients (ears)	Hematoma & Bleeding (%)	Infection (%)	Suture Reaction/Extrusion (%)	Skin Ulceration/Necrosis (%)	Hypertrophic/Keloid Scarring (%)
	Posterior SC +CM	Messner et al.	1996	31	0	3.2	9	–	3.2
	SC ± CM ± excision	Foda	1999	39	0	0	12.8	0	–
	Posterior SC +CM, posterior fascial flap	Horlock et al.	2001	51 (96)	2	0	0	0	0
	Posterior SC +CM	Mandal et al.	2006	94	5.3	1.1	3.3	0	2.1
	Posterior SC +CM, posterior fascial flap	Mandal et al.	2006	41	2.4	0	1.2	0	0
Combination	Percutaneous anterior scoring and SC, posterior conchal excision	Burres	1998	14	0	0	0	0	0
	Posterior cautery + SC ± CM	Epstein et al.	1999	60	–	–	–	0	0
	Incision, anterior scoring ± SC	Caouette-Laberge et al.	2000	500 (975)	3	0	0	0.6	0.4
	Anterior scoring + SC + CM	Yugueros and Friedland	2001	100	0	0	9.8	–	0
	Anterior scoring, excision, Kaye, CM	Erol	2001	55 (108)	0*	0*	1.8*	–	0*
	Closed anterior scoring + mattress sutures	Thomas and Fatah	2001	32 (56)	0	0	3.1	0	0
	SC + lateral conchal resection	Stucker et al.	2003	329	0.6	0.6	0.6	–	0.3
	Anterior scoring, posterior conchal incision + SC + CM	Burstein	2003	100 (200)	1	0	0	0	3
	Anterior scoring + posterior SC + CM	Kompatscher et al.	2004	14	0	–	–	–	14
	Anterior scoring + SC	Benedict and Pirwitz	2005	154 (302)	0	0.7*	9.3*	0	0.3*
	Posterior scoring + SC ± conchal excision	Scharer et al.	2007	75 (144)	1.3	0	21.3	1.3	2.7
	Closed anterior scoring + posterior SC ± conchal excision	Salgarello et al.	2007	135 (266)	6.7	0	0	1.5	2.2

SC - Scaphaconchal sutures; CM - Conchamastoid sutures
*Complication rates are reported as a percentage of ears rather than patients.

reaction to a prescribed topical antibiotic ointment. In fact, patch testing has revealed this condition to be quite common, with about 10% of people having a positive test[16]. Reactions are only slightly more frequent among neomycin-containing ointments as compared to bacitracin-containing ointments. Treatment is supportive with withdrawal and future avoidance of the offending agent. Care must be taken that this irritation does not devolve into an infectious complication. A topical steroid may be used for symptomatic relief, although contact dermatitis has more recently become a recognized complication of this drug class as well. Late skin reactions have been noted following otoplasty and these will be discussed under the topic of late complications.

Bleeding and Hematoma

The incidence of postoperative hematoma is generally reported in the low single digits and should be a relatively rare otoplasty complication if proper surgical technique is observed and tissue planes are respected. Hematomas have been reported using all otoplasty techniques, although there may be higher risk when more aggressive undermining and cutting techniques are used, especially involving the anterior auricular surface. Bleeding may begin in the immediate postoperative period following metabolism of the vasoconstrictive agents. Inciting agents may include local factors such as poor surgical technique, inadequate hemostasis, ineffective wound compression, or inadvertent trauma; and systemic factors such as hypertension or undiagnosed bleeding diatheses.

Excessive pain is the harbinger of a significant auricular hematoma, and any such complaint, especially if unilateral or asymmetrical, mandates prompt investigation and management by immediate wound inspection. If a hematoma is present, the wound should be reopened followed by evacuation of the clotted blood. Bleeding vessels should be cauterized when found, although this is unlikely. The incision should then be loosely closed over a passive drain, followed by replacement of a conforming dressing and treatment with a broad-spectrum antibiotic medication. Antimicrobial treatment is important in this setting since a hematoma may act to encourage bacterial proliferation. If left untreated for any length of time, wound infection, postinflammatory fibrosis, perichondritis, or frank chondritis may ensue with a resultant profound postoperative deformity. We have found that a loosely interrupted initial skin closure discourages blood collection under the skin, but rather allows for egress of fluids and early detection of bleeding in the early postoperative period.

Infection

Infection is infrequently observed following otoplasty (**Figure 15-1**). In a recent review[8] of otoplasty complications among 14 papers that reported them, infection was noted to occur in 0 to 5.2% of cases. It typically presents in the first postoperative week with symptoms of pain and signs of skin erythema. Purulence may be expressed from the wound edge. Contributing factors may be local, such as excessive pressure or trauma, hematoma formation, or stitch colonization; or systemic, such as immunocompromise. The risk of infection is reduced by strict observance of sterile technique and postoperative dressing care. We believe that perioperative parenteral and topical antibiotic administration, and postoperative application of antibiotic ointment to the suture line is helpful, although the benefit of antibiotic prophylaxis in a clean case is unclear. Our current regimen includes a single intravenous dose of clindamycin prior to skin incision.

Treatment of infection is by standard means of open drainage with culture of the purulent exudate, and treatment with antibiotic irrigation and systemic administration of an anti-*Pseudomonal*

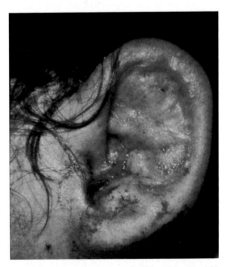

Figure 15-1. Postotoplasty cellulitis. This should be recognized quickly and treated with local wound care along with anti-Pseudomonal and anti-Staphylococcal antimicrobials in order to avoid progression.

antibiotic. Local wound care with warm compresses, wound hygiene, and topical antimicrobial agents are generally beneficial. Oral antibiotics are sufficient for a localized superficial infection; however, prompt hospital admission and intravenous multi-drug antibiotic treatment is advised for occurrences of chondritis. If necessary, devitalized tissue and eschar should be débrided to assist with resolution and further healing. If a suture otoplasty technique was used, removal of the sutures may be necessary to prevent long-term colonization. In the early postoperative period, a loss of correction will be virtually guaranteed in this setting. However, a return to surgery for the purposes of revision sometime in the future is much preferred to a protracted and complicated course of healing in a severe infection that may lead to irreversible cartilage damage if the infected suture source is left in place.

Perichondritis

Perichondritis is exceedingly rare after otoplasty, so much so that no cases were documented in a recent review of over 2000 patients[8]. This dreaded complication may evolve from an undertreated hematoma or superficial infection (**Figure 15-2**). Foreign body material in the form of retained sutures, especially of the braided variety, may promote bacterial colonization and a host inflammatory reaction that precipitates the precursor to perichondritis. In the past, episodes of perichondritis were attributed to the use of silk suture material that has proven to have less than ideal biocompatibility. This braided material was implicated in the development of perichondritis in a letter to the editor several decades ago[17]. Bull[18] does not share this sentiment, having demonstrated the safe use of white silk sutures over his 25-year otoplasty career. In contrast, he noted infectious problems with other monofilament and Teflon braided sutures.

Whatever the cause, perichondritis must be immediately recognized and quickly treated if one hopes to preserve a satisfactory outcome. Treatment should include wound exploration and culture followed by aggressive intravenous antimicrobial management with a regimen that is active against *Pseudomonas aeruginosa* and *Staphylococcus aureus*. Strong consideration should be given to hospitalization and close observation. Debridement of compromised cartilage may be necessary.

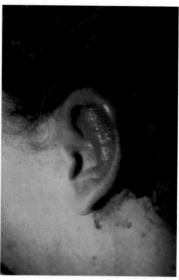

Figure 15-2. Perichondritis. This is characterized by a spreading infection that spares the lobule. The auricle is typically dark red or purple, tense, and exquisitely tender. Fever and pulse changes may be present. Consideration should be given to prompt and aggressive management with intravenous antibiotics, wound drainage, and resection of necrotic cartilage, if present.

Cartilage Necrosis

Cartilage necrosis may rarely ensue following a severe infection, perichondritis, hematoma, pressure-induced injury, or devitalization as a result of injudicious surgical dissection or cauterization (**Figure 15-3**). The most likely factors responsible are excessive use of cautery, poor surgical dissection with violation of subdermal or axial blood supply, and excessive flap compression by an overly constrictive dressing or a careless dressing causing a bent ear. Again, pain that is disproportionate to the procedure is the most common presenting complaint. Management is analogous to that for hematoma with the addition of possible skin grafting or flap advancement to cover exposed cartilage and possibly to avoid secondary chondritis. This is a terrible, although thankfully rare, complication that results in a high degree of postoperative deformity even with appropriate handling.

Skin and Wound Complications

Skin necrosis is usually attributable to flawed technique. As noted, imprudent dissection, extreme use

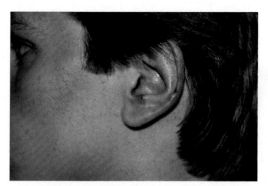

Figure 15-3. Auricular cartilage necrosis. Although exceedingly rare, this typically occurs along cartilage prominences as seen here along the helical margin, often from injudicious dressing application.

of electrocautery, and an overly compressive dressing may all predispose to this eventuality. Mercifully, frank necrosis is rare, whereas superficial skin ulceration is slightly more common. Nevertheless, this problem is still reported in less than 1% of otoplasty cases. Skin ulceration from a tight dressing will tend to occur over cartilage prominences and can usually be treated conservatively with the expectation of a good outcome.

Wound dehiscence is another uncommon, although known complication of otoplasty. This trouble tends to occur when too much skin is excised, placing excessive tension on the closure. Dehiscence may also ensue when appropriate splinting by suture techniques or other methods is inadequate to maintain the desired auricular contour and the skin closure is inappropriately relied upon to maintain the correction. Infection, hematoma, and injury to the skin flap may also constitute predisposing factors.

Late Complications

Late complications manifest sometime in the weeks to months following the procedure and may be more subtle or gradual in presentation. Late manifestations, such as recurrence of the deformity, that primarily constitute aesthetic concerns are more properly referred to as undesirable aesthetic sequelae rather than true complications. These will be addressed in the next chapter.

Suture Complications

A range of problems can arise secondary to suture utilization in otoplasty (**Figure 15-4**).

Suturerelated complications may relate to specific faults in technique. For example, incorrect suture placement may be responsible for anterior displacement of the conchal cartilage leading to external auditory canal occlusion. Similarly, overzealous scaphaconchal stitch tightening may lead to antihelical overcorrection and a hidden helix deformity.

However, when we talk about suture complications in otoplasty, we are really speaking of problems related to the presence of the suture material itself. Resorbable sutures are a common source of localized skin inflammation and stitch abscess formation in the short term. Permanent sutures, on the other hand, especially those of the braided variety, more frequently precipitate development of indolent infections or foreign-body granulomas. Monofilament sutures, while less reactive, have a greater tendency to slippage, a feature that may negatively affect the cosmetic result. A majority of studies, though not all, showing a high rate of suture extrusion have used Mersilene or other braided sutures (**see Table 15-1**). Rigg[19] reported 11 Mersilene suture granulomas in 70 patients (15.7%), prompting a switch to nylon suture for construction of the antihelix in the remaining patients in this series. Maniglia et al.,[20] reported one case of extrusion in 42 ears using nylon while Goode and Proffit[7] experienced this complication in two of 126 ears using Dacron. Mersilene sutures have been used by the senior author for the past 20 years with excellent results and a low incidence of suture complications[21]. Mustardé[22] himself published a series of 600 ears treated over 20 years in which only 1% developed sinus tracts and silk suture rejection, and loss of correction was severe enough to warrant revision in 1.7%. The classic Mustardé suture technique has not proven as successfully reproducible in the hands of others.

Suture extrusion is usually a late phenomenon after otoplasty and, as such, typically does not have a negative effect on the cosmetic outcome. In these instances, removal of the offending suture is curative, although premature suture removal may predispose to loss of correction. Thus, this procedure may be postponed for several weeks to months to allow for some fibrosis and maintenance of correction to occur. We have found that patients generally do not experience recurrence if sutures are removed more than about 8 weeks postoperatively. Scaphoconchal Mustardé sutures are more likely than conchomastoid sutures to extrude, as they are

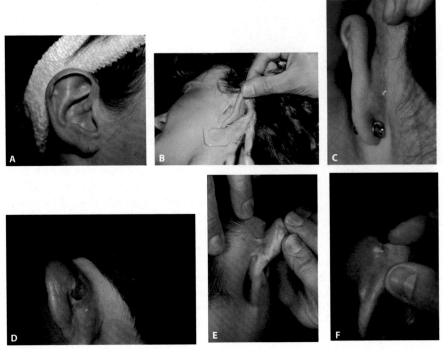

Figure 15-4. Suture complications following otoplasty. (A) Suture visibility. (B) Suture erosion. (C) Suture extrusion. (D) Suture granuloma or ulceration. (E) Suture banding. (F) Suture pull through.

located in a more superficial subcutaneous plane, especially at the superior pole. If placed too distal relative to the antihelical fold, these sutures may be seen to 'bowstring' across the gap, causing both an aesthetic and functional deformity. These are more likely to be functionally problematic for patients who wear eyeglasses. The tendency for stitch banding is exacerbated in the setting of excessive skin excision where there is a tense skin closure and poor suture coverage.

Suture visibility and overlying skin reaction or erosion may also occur when there is insufficient soft tissue coverage. This is especially true when knots are placed from an anterior approach. Horlock and colleagues[23] recommend routine use of a posterior fascial flap to improve suture coverage. In their experience, this addition has essentially eliminated the problems of suture extrusion, visibility, and banding. Romo et al.,[24] reported on their use of a medially based postauricular skin flap approach to a cartilage-sparing otoplasty. They found this method beneficial in 25 patients studied in that the desired skin excision did not need to be estimated preoperatively. By reserving a more conservative skin excision for the procedure's conclusion, they were able to more

accurately assess the degree of residual skin required for ample tissue coverage without tension, thereby minimizing the risk of suture extrusion.

Dysesthesias

Sensory abnormalities following otoplasty may include the experience of protracted pain or hyperesthesia, hypoesthesia, or paresthesia. Persistent sensory deficits and dysfunction following otoplasty have been thought by many to be quite rare. A very comprehensive, long-term survey in a large series of patients suggests otherwise. Caouette-Laberge and colleagues[25] sent a questionnaire to patients to elicit their concerns at least two years after surgery. Residual pain was reported by 5.7%, persistent hypoesthesia by 3.9%, and sensitivity to cold and touch by 7.5% of patients. Similarly, 9.7% of patients in another study[26] acknowledged having lasting hyperesthesia when questioned directly. While injury to the robust sensory nerve supply of the auricle may give rise to these symptoms initially, they are usually expected to resolve spontaneously over several months. Persistent pain and hyperesthesia may result from failure of terminal sensory fibers to regenerate

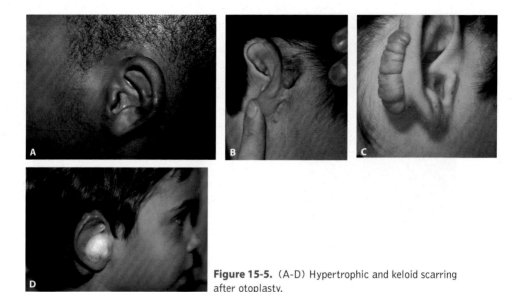

Figure 15-5. (A-D) Hypertrophic and keloid scarring after otoplasty.

properly or from the development of faulty central feedback mechanisms. In a small cadre of patients, lingering cold temperature insensitivity may present a very real risk of frostbite following otoplasty, likely owing to disruption of auricular blood supply. Patients should be made aware of such possibilities and be advised to take appropriate precautionary measures.

Unacceptable Scarring

Hypertrophic scarring or keloid formation seldom occurs after otoplasty, with all studies noting an incidence of less than 5%. Keloid scarring occurs almost exclusively in susceptible individuals of African, Asian, or Scandinavian descent. Younger patients are also more vulnerable, especially in the setting of postauricular incisions (**Figure 15-5**). A personal or family history of keloid scarring is understandably the most essential risk factor, and this history should be obtained preoperatively so that proper counseling may be offered. Preventive modalities include avoidance of excessive wound-closing tension and minimization of tissue trauma or infection.

If they develop, hypertrophic scars and keloids are treated as in other locations. Hypertrophic scars may be monitored for spontaneous regression, although most surgeons tend to treat them with serial injections of small volumes of triamcinolone acetate (10 to 40 mg/mL) every few weeks followed by exci-

sion for those failing to respond favorably. Silicone sheeting may play a role in flattening of the scar. Keloids are treated in a similar fashion although they tend to be recalcitrant to typical therapies. More aggressive handling may be necessary in the form of serial excision, laser energy vaporization, or low-dose external beam radiation therapy. Some authors recommend leaving a rim of keloid scar behind during excision to discourage recurrence of abnormal tissue healing at the wound's periphery. Since keloids can be particularly problematic to treat, every effort should be made to avoid them during commission of the initial surgery.

Other Skin and Subcutaneous Sequelae

Additional skin conditions may occur long after the ear has healed (**Figure 15-6**). Idiopathic dermatitis affecting the ear has been reported by up to 9.8% of patients in one long-term survey[25]. In this survey, 'skin lesions' were reported to occur within the newly created folds on the front and back of the ear. The skin condition most frequently noted was that of eczema. This condition constitutes a post-traumatic dermatitis, an idiopathic phenomenon whose existence has been well documented in other areas. Intertrigo, a superficial fungal infection of the skin folds, developed secondarily in a number of patients. This problem typically occurs in moist skin

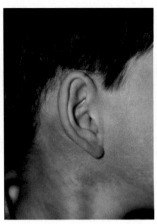

Figure 15-6. Postototplasty periauricular dermatitis.

folds elsewhere in the body, and may likewise be seen more frequently when there is overcorrection of the prominent ear with creation of excessively deep folds and furrows.

Epidermal and subdermal inclusion cysts may also occur with relative frequency following otoplasty (**Figure 15-7**). These can usually be attributed to microscopic entrapment and implantation of epithelial elements into the dermis or subdermis during healing. This may occur within an otoplasty scar. It is a more realistic risk of small access and incisionless otoplasty techniques if great care is not taken to pass the suture needle back through exactly the same point through which it exited. If present, an epidermal cyst is easily managed by simple enucleation and excision.

Dermatologic sequelae do not feature prominently in the literature as potential long-term consequences of otoplasty. This almost certainly is not because they occur infrequently, as a 10% incidence

of postoperative skin reactions as seen above is not negligible and must surely exist in other series. Related symptoms may not be of sufficient gravity to raise concerns, although we would postulate that they are probably bothersome to affected patients. They most likely occur with sufficient delay to escape detection by surgeons who have probably discharged patients from their care by the time of onset of these conditions. The most likely explanation is that such occurrences, whether by virtue of temporal dissociation or due to other factors, do not elicit an association with the surgery until patients are explicitly asked about them. For this reason, long-term open studies of patient outcomes with cosmetic facial procedures are invaluable and investigators who undertake such efforts are to be commended for them. Without studies such as these, we really do not know what we are missing.

In this chapter, we reviewed the incidence of true surgical complications among current English-literature otoplasty articles encompassing large patient series utilizing various surgical techniques. The limitations of such comparisons have been duly noted owing to the highly subjective nature in which complications are defined by specific authors, and to the reporting and selection bias inherent to many series. Nevertheless, the rates of near-term wound and bleeding complications appear to be on the whole greater among cartilage-splitting techniques, while the regular incidence of suture complications is obviously unique to cartilage-sparing suture techniques. In the next and final chapter, we will highlight the comparative prevalence of aesthetic consequences among the foremost otoplasty techniques, including loss of correction and the need for revision surgery. We will further characterize the origins of the most frequent aesthetic otoplasty pitfalls and disclose surgical pearls for their prevention.

References

1. Jeffery S. Complications following correction of prominent ears: an audit review of 122 cases. *Br J Plast Surg* 52:588, 1999.
2. Tan KH. Long-term survey of prominent ear surgery: a comparison of two methods. *Br J Plast Surg* 39(2): 270–3, 1986.
3. Scharer SA, Farrior EH, Farrior RT. Retrospective analysis of the Farrior technique for otoplasty. *Arch Facial Plast Surg* 9:167–73, 2007.
4. Calder JC, Naasan A. Morbidity of otoplasty: a retrospective review of 562 consecutive cases. *Br J Plast Surg* 47:170, 1994.

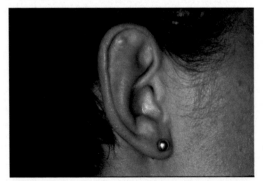

Figure 15-7. Subdermal cyst or granuloma secondary to use of permanent suture in otoplasty.

5. McDowell AJ. Goals in otoplasty for protruding ears. *Plast Reconstr Surg* 41:17–27, 1968.
6. Wright WK. Otoplasty goals and principles. *Arch Otolaryngol* 92:568–72, 1970.
7. Goode RL, Proffitt SD, Rafaty FM. Complications of otoplasty. *Arch Otolaryngol* 91(4):352–5, 1970.
8. Zavod MB, Chen T, Adamson PA. Complications of Otoplasty, Ch. 59. In: Eisele D, Smith R, eds. Complications in Head and Neck Surgery, 2nd edition. *Mosby,* In Press.
9. Honkavaara P, Pyykko I: Effects of atropine and scopolamine on bradycardia and emetic symptoms in otoplasty. *Laryngoscope* 109(1):108–112, 1999.
10. Paxton D, Taylor RH, Gallagher TM, et al: Post-operative emesis following otoplasty in children. *Anaesthesia* 50(12):1083–1085, 1995.
11. Lancaster JL, Jones TM, Kay AR, McGeorge DD. Pediatric day-case otoplasty: local versus general anaesthetic. *Surgeon* 1(2):96–8, 2003.
12. Ferraro GA, Corcione A, Nicoletti G, Rossano F, Perrotta A, D'Andrea F. Blepharoplasty and otoplasty: comparative sedation with remifentanil, propofol, and midazolam. *Aesthetic Plast Surg* 29(3):181–3, 2005.
13. Pavlin DJ, Chen C, Penazola DA, Polissar NL, Buckley FP. Pain as a factor complicating recovery and discharge after ambulatory surgery. *Anesth Analg* 95(3): 627–34, 2002.
14. Cregg N, Conway F, Casey W. Analgesia after otoplasty: regional nerve blockade vs local anesthetic infiltration of the ear. *Can J Anaesth* 43(2):141–7, 1996.
15. Koeppe T, Constantinescu MA, Schneider J, Gubisch W. Current trends in local anesthesia in cosmetic plastic surgery of the head and neck: results of a German national survey and observation on the use of ropivacaine. *Plast Reconstr Surg* 115(6):1723–30, 2005.
16. Wetter DA, Davis MD, Yiannias JA, et al: Patch test results from the Mayo Clinic Contact Dermatitis Group, 1998–2000. *J Am Acad Dermatol* 53(3):416–421, 2005.
17. Zohar Y. Otoplasty. *Arch Otolaryngol* 96:187, 1972.
18. Bull TR. Otoplasty: Mustardé technique. *Facial Plast Surg* 10(3):267–76, 1994.
19. Rigg BM. Suture materials in otoplasty. *Plast Reconstr Surg* 63:409–10, 1979.
20. Maniglia AJ, Maniglia JJ, Witten BR. Otoplasty: an eclectic technique. *Laryngoscope* 1977;87:1359–68, 1977.
21. Adamson PA, McGraw BL, Tropper GJ: Otoplasty: Critical review of clinical results. *Laryngoscope* 101(8): 883–88, 1991.
22. Mustardé JC. Results of otoplasty by the author's method. In: Goldwyn RM, ed. Long-term results in plastic and reconstructive surgery. *Boston, Little Brown,* p. 146, 1980.
23. Horlock N, Misra A, Gault DT. The postauricular fascial flap as an adjunct to Mustardé and Furnas-type otoplasty. *Plast Reconstr Surg* 108(6):1487–90, 2001.
24. Romo T 3rd, Sclafani AP, Shapiro AL. Otoplasty using the postauricular skin flap technique. *Arch Otolaryngol Head Neck Surg* 120(10):1146–50, 1994.
25. Caouette-Laberge L, Guay N, Bortoluzzi P, Belleville C. Otoplasty: anterior scoring technique and results in 500 cases. *Plast Reconstr Surg* 105(2):504–15, 2000.
26. Messner AH, Crysdale WS: Otoplasty: Clinical protocol and long-term results. *Arch Otolaryngol Head Neck Surg* 122(7):773–77, 1996.

16

AESTHETIC PITFALLS IN OTOPLASTY

PETER A. ADAMSON, MD, FRCSC, FACS AND
JASON A. LITNER, MD, FRCSC

Introduction

In the preceding chapter, we characterized the surgical complications that may occur following otoplasty. Despite the potential for such problems, patient satisfaction is uniformly high for this procedure (see Table 16-1). In a review of various otoplasty techniques[1], the rate of patient satisfaction was over 90% for all series studied. Not surprisingly, surgeons were somewhat more critical of their own results, with a dissatisfaction rate of 7.7% compared to 4.3% of patients.

The mere absence of a surgical complication does not, in and of itself, guarantee a pleasing outcome. Aesthetic shortfalls have occurred in all studies regardless of the particular otoplasty technique used. Numerous technical errors must be consciously circumvented in order to secure a balanced and harmonious auricular contour and proportion. In this final chapter, we will discuss the technical failures that may result in undesirable aesthetic sequelae for it is these, more than minor surgical complications, which most often engender long-term patient discontent with the procedure. Moreover, we will emphasize measures that should be taken to minimize the threat of such complications.

General Aesthetic Pitfalls

Patient Dissatisfaction

This is a less common complication following otoplasty as compared to most facial aesthetic procedures. Satisfaction with the surgical outcome relates as much to the patient's preoperative expectations as it does to superlative technical performance. Selection of a patient for otoplasty requires his or her understanding of the complexities of this operation and acceptance of realistic possible outcomes. The explanation of risks should be tailored to the patient's particular situation rather than comprise a simple generalization. Not all patients who have experienced a complication are ultimately dissatisfied with their outcomes. Most patients are willing to accept the possibility of a complication. If patients sense that the surgeon has and will continue to listen to them and to do whatever is reasonable to assure their happiness, they will generally harbor positive feelings towards the surgeon. In fact, if handled always with delicacy and respect for the patient's wellbeing at heart, many such patients will go on to become the surgeon's greatest advocates and supporters.

Similarly, a good technical result from the surgeon's perspective may not be considered desirable by the patient if it failed to meet expectations. A comprehensive preoperative discussion should emphasize the probability of an improved, but less than perfect, result as it is nearly impossible to achieve perfect auricular symmetry. Following otoplasty, slight asymmetries within 2 to 3 mm upon side-to-side comparison are considered acceptable and well within the normal range of experience. The great majority of patients are content with such a

TABLE 16-1 Rates of patient and surgeon satisfaction by otoplasty technique, author, year, and number of patients

Technique	Method	Author	Year	No. of patients (ears)	Patient Satisfaction (%)	Surgeon Satisfaction (%)
Cartilage Cutting	Pitanguy Island flap ± conchal excision	Bartkowski et al.	2001	80	–	85
	Anterior skin + conchal excision, posterior mattress sutures	Bauer et al.	2002	47 (87)	100	100
	Cartilage tubing, anterior scoring	Peker and Celikoz	2002	178 (343)	95	–
	Posterior incision + mattress sutures	Panettiere et al.	2004	33	–	95
	Cartilage tubing ± conchal excision	Kompatscher et al.	2004	14	100	43
Cartilage Scoring	Anterior scoring ± conchal excision	Nordzell	2000	80 (160)	96	76
	Posterior scoring + mattress sutures	Panettiere et al.	2004	30	–	95
	Anterior scoring	Mandal et al.	2006	68	86.7	–
Cartilage Suturing	SC	Minderjahn et al.	1980	135	–	88
	SC	Attwood and Evans	1985	52	100	–
	Modified SC	Koch et al.	1991	340	91.4	–
	Posterior SC + CM	Adamson et al.	1991	62 (119)	95	95
	Posterior SC + CM	Vuyk et al.	1994	62 (117)	–	92
	Posterior SC + CM	Messner et al.	1996	31	94	94
	Posterior SC + CM	Mandal et al.	2006	94	89.3	–
	Posterior SC + CM, posterior fascial flap	Mandal et al.	2006	41	97.4	–
Combination	Posterior scoring + Kaye sutures	Pilz et al.	1995	167	90	–
	Percutaneous anterior scoring and SC, posterior conchal excision	Burres	1998	14	100	–
	Anterior scoring, SC + posterior CM	Dechamboux et al.	2000	368	83	–
	Incision, anterior scoring ± SC	Caouette-Laberge et al.	2000	500 (975)	94.8	96
	Closed anterior scoring + mattress sutures	Thomas and Fatah	2001	32 (56)	95	–
	Posterior mattress sutures ± scoring	Vital and Printza	2002	86	94	96
	Anterior scoring + posterior SC + CM	Kompatscher et al.	2004	14	100	93
	Closed anterior scoring + posterior SC ± conchal excision	Salgarello et al.	2007	135 (266)	95	95

SC- Scaphaconchal sutures; CM- Conchamastoid sutures

result and is not interested in revision in the presence of mild asymmetry. Patients can usually be reassured of this fact; however, occasional revisions may be undertaken when considered appropriate.

Residual Deformity or Reprotrusion

Residual deformity and reprotrusion are, by far, the two most common postoperative otoplasty complications encountered[2,3], with reported rates ranging from 0% to 57% (**see Table 16-2**). Residual deformity refers to undercorrection that is observable shortly after the procedure, whereas reprotrusion speaks more toward a technical breakdown that causes an acceptable result to deteriorate over time. This usually becomes apparent within several months following the procedure. Since these problems are sometimes lumped in together or are otherwise indistinguishable in the literature, they will be discussed collectively.

Undercorrection leading to a residual deformity may occur using any technique. However, it may be encountered more frequently when a cartilage-sparing approach is utilized in the setting of a strong, inflexible cartilaginous framework whose spring has not been appropriately weakened. Reprotrusion is most frequently seen using cartilage-sparing techniques and, if related to technical deficiencies, will usually present in the first several postoperative months. This occurs more often in cartilage-suture techniques wherein the intrinsic cartilage tension prevails over the tightening effect provided by the sutures. Technical flaws may include improper location of sutures, placement of too few sutures resulting in excessive tension and pull-through of one or more sutures, or failure to overcorrect at the time of the operation. Failure to 'bite' the perichondrial layers is most often implicated as a source of suture pull-through.

There may be some anatomic predisposition to loss of correction in cartilage-sparing otoplasty. Less commonly, technical failure may not relate to antihelical suture placement at all but rather to failure to obtain sufficient conchal setback. Many authors[3–6] have reported a preponderance of suture failures to occur at the superior pole. Some authors[7] have noted the tendency for slight reprotrusion in all suture otoplasties, and have advocated for the routine addition of scoring techniques. Others feel that adjusting accordingly by routine overcorrection provides a satisfactory solution to correct for the inevitable reprotrusion that can be as much as 40% of the original correction[8]. In contrast, Stenström and Heftner[9] reported that, in their experience with an anterior cartilage-scoring otoplasty technique, the correction obtained on the operative table proved to be a stable and dependable result. These differences of opinion may reflect the probability of suture slippage in suture-dependent otoplasties versus more reliable cartilage remodeling attainable with cartilage-scoring and cartilage-cutting techniques.

Furnas[10] has distinguished suture failure according to principal causes, whether from intrinsic mechanics, such as excessive cartilage spring, or extrinsic stresses, such as those applied by an unfavorable dressing or sleeping position. In fact, associated external trauma was a noteworthy contributing factor in approximately half of the cases of loss of correction in our series[3]. Loss of correction, especially at the superior pole, is not simply a phenomenon of cartilage-sparing techniques. Farrior and colleagues[11] noted a reprotrusion rate of 22.3% using a combination technique. Various authors have alternately correlated reprotrusion risk with a short helical diameter[4] or a tall vertical auricular height[12]. Incidence of this complication may be lessened in a suture technique by careful placement of sutures with attainment of adequate purchase on the anterior perichondrium to avert suture pull-through, and by placement of conchotemporal tension-relieving sutures to help anchor the correction[3].

Interestingly, at least two authors have correlated the incidence of reprotrusion with the surgeon's experience level. Calder and Naasan[6] noted that 73% of residual deformities in their series could be attributed to an error in the design of the cartilage manipulation. Caouette-Laberge and colleagues[12] reported a more than 3-fold incidence of late complications when the ear was operated upon by a resident compared to a senior surgeon. Therefore, the supervising surgeon should carefully consider the level of experience of a trainee during intraoperative planning and execution. Minderjahn and colleagues[13] reported a strong association between reprotrusion and cartilage thickness. In their series, cases experiencing relapse all occurred in ears exceeding 3.1 mm in width at the fossa triangularis or 3.4 mm at the cavum concha. As noted previously, surgeons may need to consider more powerful cartilage-weakening maneuvers when faced with these cases.

Overcorrection

Overcorrection is a relatively frequent finding in those series that record it, and appears to be independent of the preferred otoplasty technique. This rate varies depending on the operating surgeon. Stenström and Heftner[9] reported some degree of overcorrection in 25% of their patients after a cartilage-scoring otoplasty. This phenomenon tended towards increasing frequency in the ears that were most prominent preoperatively. Minderjahn

TABLE 16-2 Comparison of aesthetic sequelae by otoplasty technique, author, year, and number of patients

Technique	Method	Author	Year	No. of patients (ears)	Residual/ Recurrent Protrusion (%)	Overcorrection (%)	Asymmetry (%)	Contour Irregularity (%)	Revision Rate (%)
Cartilage Cutting	Pitanguy Island flap ± conchal excision	Bartkowski et al.	2001	80	–	–	5	–	3.8
	Anterior skin + conchal excision, posterior mattress sutures	Bauer et al.	2002	47 (87)	6.4	–	–	–	6.4
	Cartilage tubing, anterior scoring	Peker and Celikoz	2002	178 (343)	–	–	6.7	–	0
	Posterior incision + mattress sutures	Panettiere et al.	2004	33	4	–	–	92	–
	Cartilage tubing ± conchal excision	Kompatscher et al.	2004	14	57	7	86	33	–
	Pitanguy Island flap + SC ± conchal excision	Werdin et al.	2007	278 (551)	4*	–	–	0.9*	4*
Cartilage Scoring	Incision + anterior scoring	Chongchet	1963	21	10	–	–	–	–
	Anterior scoring	Tan	1986	101	14.3	–	–	–	–
	Incision + anterior scoring	Calder and Naasan	1994	562	8	–	11	–	11
	Anterior scoring ± SC	Jeffery	1999	122	12.7	–	–	–	3.3
	Anterior scoring + SC	Azuara	2000	(100)	0*	0*	1*	0*	1*
	Anterior scoring ± conchal excision	Nordzell	2000	80 (160)	6.2	6.2	2.5	5	3.8
	Percutaneous anterior scoring + SC	Bulstrode et al.	2003	114 (214)	6.1	–	0	0	2.6
	Anterior scoring + SC	Nolst Trenité	2004	65	4.6	–	–	6.2	0
	Posterior scoring + mattress sutures	Panettiere et al.	2004	30	2	–	–	0	–
	Anterior abrasion ± CM	Di Mascio et al.	2004	40 (75)	5	–	–	–	–
	Anterior scoring	Raunig	2005	(302)	1*	–	0*	0*	0.7*
	Anterior scoring	Mandal et al.	2006	68	11	–	–	1.4	8.8
	Anterior scoring + CM	Bhatti and Donavan	2007	34 (68)	0	–	–	–	0
Cartilage Suturing	SC + CM	Rigg	1979	101	2	–	–	–	–
	SC	Minderjahn et al.	1980	135	13.3	39	40	–	–
	SC	Attwood and Evans	1985	52	0	–	–	–	0
	SC	Tan	1986	45	24.4	–	–	–	–
	Modified SC	Koch et al.	1991	340	17	–	–	0	–
	Posterior SC + CM	Adamson et al.	1991	62 (119)	6.6*	0*	0*	0*	6.6*

Posterior SC + CM	Vuyk et al.	1994	62 (117)	5.1*	2.5*	–	–	1.7*
Posterior SC + CM	Messner et al.	1996	31	6.4	–	6.4	–	6.4
SC ± CM ± excision	Foda	1999	39	5.1	–	–	–	–
Posterior SC + CM, posterior fascial flap	Horlock et al.	2001	51 (96)	11.8	–	–	–	2
Posterior SC + CM	Mandal et al.	2006	94	8	–	–	0	6
Posterior SC + CM, posterior fascial flap	Mandal et al.	2006	41	4.8	–	–	0	3.6
Percutaneous anterior scoring and SC, posterior conchal excision	Burres	1998	14	28.6	–	–	–	0
Combination								
Posterior cautery + SC ± CM	Epstein et al.	1999	60	10	–	–	–	10
Incision, anterior scoring ± SC	Caouette-Laberge et al.	2000	500 (975)	4.4	0.4	5.6	–	1.2
Anterior scoring + SC + CM	Yugueros and Friedland	2001	100	3.6	–	0	–	3.1
Anterior scoring, excision, Kaye, CM	Erol	2001	55 (108)	3.6*	3.6*	0*	–	1.9*
Closed anterior scoring + mattress sutures	Thomas and Fatah	2001	32 (56)	3.1	–	–	–	0
SC + lateral conchal resection	Stucker et al.	2003	329	0	–	0	–	0.6
Anterior scoring, posterior conchal incision + SC + CM	Burstein	2003	100 (200)	8	–	0	–	8
Anterior scoring + posterior SC + CM	Kompatscher et al.	2004	14	36	14	50	33	–
Anterior scoring + SC	Benedict and Pirwitz	2005	154 (302)	9.9*	–	–	–	9.9*
Posterior scoring + SC ± conchal excision	Scharer et al.	2007	75 (144)	22.3	1.5	–	–	12
Closed anterior scoring + posterior SC ± conchal excision	Salgarello et al.	2007	135 (266)	3	–	–	–	0

SC – Scaphaconchal sutures; CM – Conchamastoid sutures
*complication rates are reported as a percentage of ears rather than patients

and associates[13] experienced overcorrection in as much as 39% of their patients undergoing a Mustardé otoplasty. This finding usually occurred in those operated on by experienced surgeons who would normally achieve superior antihelical configuration and upper pole medialization. As has been our experience, such overcorrection was generally considered attractive by the patients and their families.

Interaural Asymmetry

Precise interaural replication of all otoplasty maneuvers, including the site and vector of pull of suture placement and the location and extent of excisions, is critical to maintaining superior interaural symmetry. Failure to attend to this need may result in an unacceptably high degree of postoperative asymmetry. Despite obvious efforts to the contrary, interaural asymmetry has been seen to occur with relative frequency after otoplasty. In their elaborate statistical analysis of their results, Minderjahn et al.[13] found objective asymmetrical correction in 40% of their patients. A difference in auricular protrusion of 2 mm or less usually went unnoticed by patients. Asymmetry was more easily noticed in lobular protrusion and less so when it involved the superior pole. Interestingly, in one large series Caouette-Laberge et al.[12] reported a rate of asymmetry of 5.6% on reevaluation up to 64 months after surgery. A survey mailed to patients, however, revealed a self-reported incidence of interaural asymmetry in 18.4% of patients more than 2 years after surgery. Therefore, it appears that patients may have a different view of asymmetry than do their corresponding surgeons. An alternate explanation is that asymmetry worsens with time as these surveys were conducted much later than the follow-up screenings. This finding underscores the importance of long-term follow-up studies to evaluate evolving postoperative changes.

Nevertheless, most authors note that asymmetry is not often reason enough for a patient to request revision surgery. This may be because both ears can be viewed together during interpersonal communication only within about 15 degrees of the midline. Even then, only differences in lateral auricular projection are visible from this stance. This may account for the fact that asymmetry is not a commonly featured complaint after otoplasty. Exceptions do exist, however, with at least one series[6] reporting that 11% of patients either had or were awaiting operative revision to improve their auricular symmetry.

Frequent reevaluation and comparisons of both ears throughout the procedure will increase the probability of attaining a natural and symmetrical result. Manushakian et al.[14] described the novel use of prone positioning of the patient in more than 100 cases in order to aid in constant comparison between ears without the need for frequent repositioning. Final suture knot tightening should be postponed until the surgeon is assured of precise and correct suture placement. As discussed earlier, when prominauris is present only unilaterally, the patient should be advised of the possibility of achieving greater balance if both ears are operated upon despite the relative normalcy of the uninvolved side. When both ears are affected, most authors have found that correction of the most affected ear first enhances the surgeon's ability to achieve acceptable symmetry because smaller corrections of the least affected ear are easier to control secondarily. In general, achievement of interaural symmetry within 2 to 3 millimeters is considered to fall within acceptable norms. In the preoperative consultation, the patient should be apprised of any pre-existing asymmetries, as these are difficult to correct entirely.

Operative Revision

Revision surgery is arguably the most definitive determinant of success or failure for any aesthetic procedure. By definition, an operative revision indicates that either the patient or caregiver is dissatisfied enough to choose another procedure over acceptance of a suboptimal result. Revision rates in the otoplasty literature have a wide variance from 0% to 24% of patients although variations in the recording and reporting of revisions, among other complications, make direct comparisons unfeasible. The most common reason for revision surgery in most series is undercorrection or reprotrusion, followed by aesthetic sequelae such as notching or cartilaginous irregularities. By contrast, patients tend to tolerate slight overcorrection far better than equivalent undercorrection. In general, reported rates for revision surgery in most series are lower than the rates of patients having unsatisfactory cosmetic results. It becomes apparent, then, that either the patient or the surgeon is often willing to accept a certain degree of irregularity rather than demand a revision procedure.

Specific Technical Aesthetic Pitfalls

Walter and Nolst Trenité[15] have noted the most common postoperative deformities found after inadequately applied otoplasty techniques to be:

- An obliterated postauricular sulcus,
- Irregularities or a sharp antihelical vault,
- A 'telephone ear' deformity,
- A protruding lobule,
- An obliterated external ear canal, and
- Postperichondritis deformations

In the following descriptions, we will characterize these and other notable, and preventable, aesthetic deformities.

Telephone Ear Deformity

This deformity arises from overzealous antihelical suturing, conchal setback, or postauricular skin excision within the middle third of the auricle, causing a relative protrusion of the superior and inferior poles (**Figure 16-1**). Insufficient correction or loss of correction at the superior and inferior poles may also present with this appearance. Caution should be exercised to avoid such overcorrection. Many authors recommend a dumbbell-shaped skin excision in order to avoid excessive tension within the mid-pole. This type of skin excision ensures that enough skin is preserved in the mid-pole to avert this deformity. We have found that a conservative fusiform

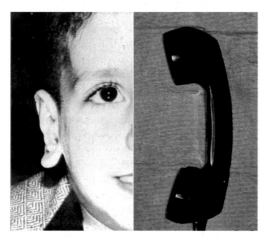

Figure 16-1. Telephone ear deformity. Note the protrusive superior pole and lobule and over-corrected middle third.

skin excision in combination with tying down of the mid-pole sutures last during antihelical suture contouring may significantly diminish the likelihood of this deformity.

To correct this deformity, a total revision procedure is necessary. Walter and Nolst Trenité[15] advocate a posterior approach with complete freeing of the posterior cartilaginous surface. Cartilage reshaping is performed by increasing its tension or by removal of excess cartilage. Deficient antihelical cartilage in the mid-pole is treated by external mattress suture plication of a cartilaginous graft in a subcutaneous pocket created along the anterior antihelical surface.

Reverse Telephone Ear Deformity

This deformity occurs in the opposing scenario, wherein middle third prominence persists, usually resulting from a failure to recognize or adequately address excessive mid-conchal wall height. In this situation, retropositioning is attempted but not accomplished by isolated antihelical folding without attendant conchal setback. A characteristic conchal misalignment results from this scenario.

Vertical Post Deformity

This moniker refers to a distinctive exaggerated vertical scaphal folding and buckled helical rim caused by Mustardé suture placement in a vertical rather than oblique orientation. The antihelix, in this scenario, loses its natural curvature and, instead, takes on a vertical course. This deformity may be avoided by judicious placement of a suitable number of sutures in an oblique orientation conforming to the natural curvilinear arc of the helix and antihelix.

Hidden Helix Deformity

More common even than conchal overcorrection, as noted below, is the condition in which the concha is undercorrected and compensatory over-corrective antihelical folding is undertaken (**Figure 16-2**). This presents a situation in which the antihelix is the most laterally protruding structure on frontal view, thereby yielding the aptly named "hidden helix" defect. This predicament is forestalled by preliminary conchal setback followed by assessment of the need for antihelical furling, which is usually less than initially projected. Overcorrection of the antihelix may

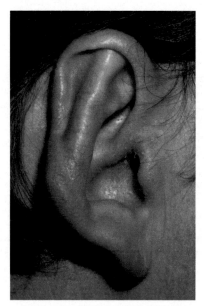

Figure 16-2. Hidden helix deformity resulting from overcorrection of the antihelical fold.

also be prevented by tying down the middle third sutures last, as is our preference.

Antihelical Creasing or Puckering

Mustardé sutures that are too closely placed, span too narrow a segment of cartilage, or are too tightly knotted will produce an abrupt crease rather than the desired gentle roll of the antihelix. Similarly, overly large bites of greater than 6 mm may generate areas of puckering or rippling within the scapha. Careful attention to suture placement will forego the potential for such sequelae. Similar abnormalities may result from imprudent cartilage-splitting techniques (**Figure 16-3**).

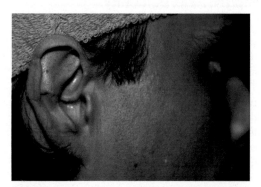

Figure 16-3. Puckering of the antihelical cartilage by imprudent design of cartilage-cutting techniques.

Antihelical Malposition

Creation of the new antihelical fold in an unnaturally anterior position relative to the helix will yield a scaphoid fossa that is too wide for the ear. Regardless of the technique used to recreate the antihelix, care must be taken in the design of its placement relative to the helical furl (**Figure 16-4**).

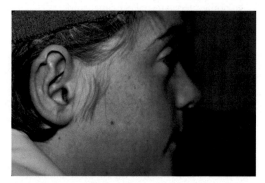

Figure 16-4. Antihelical malposition. Poorly designed antihelical cartilage-cutting contouring maneuvers result in an unnatural antihelical relief.

Auricular Ridges or Sharp Edges

Full thickness incisional cartilage-cutting techniques significantly destabilize the auricular cartilage and are subject to a far greater probability of sharply visible cartilaginous edges and anterior surface ridges (**Figure 16-5**). Changes in tensional forces with healing over time predispose to frequent occurrences of these visible step deformities, especially along the antihelical fold, in patients subjected to these techniques. These ears look very unnatural and are often very disconcerting to the affected patients. Therefore, we confine our cutting techniques to finely feathered abrasions or scoring of the anterior antihelical surface only in the rare instance of a markedly stiff cartilage. In this way, we avoid visible contour irregularities. We have not found our capacity for attainment of reliably satisfactory surgical correction to be adversely affected by this viewpoint.

If present, small irregularities may be smoothed by simple curettage with a House curette, according to Walter[15]. This may be accessed via a small incision at the ear lobe or in the superior crus. If there is disfiguring tissue loss or a significantly sharp cartilaginous edge, this may be treated by creation of a subcutaneous pocket over the affected area and interposition of an overlay camouflage graft.

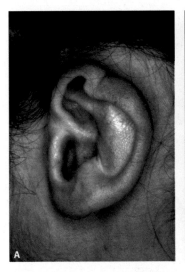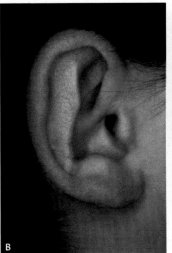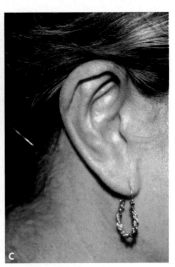

Figure 16-5. Auricular contour abnormalities secondary to poorly planned cartilage-splitting techniques. (A) Helical notching. (B) Sharp antihelical ridge. (C) Antihelical contour irregularity.

Temporalis fascia or cartilage from the concha is ideal for this purpose, though the use of Gore-Tex has also been described.

Retroauricular Sulcus Obliteration

Excessive conchal bowl resection or skin excision may sometimes result in extreme flattening or recession of the concha, giving the ear a very unnatural "glued down" appearance. At times, excessive furling of the antihelix may aggravate this appearance. Nolst Trenité[16] has suggested leaving at least 1 cm of skin on either side of the designed skin excision in order to ensure preservation of an adequate retro-auricular sulcus. When faced with prospective revision of an obliterated sulcus, Walter[15] advises use of a zigzag skin incision with suturing of the ensuing flaps point-to-point to widen the postauricular sulcus (**Figure 16-6**). The intervening raw areas thus created are covered by full thickness skin grafts. The advantage of this technique over skin grafting alone is the diminished tendency for skin contraction. The patient is advised to wear a spacer device similar to a behind-the-ear hearing aid for a period of 3 months to maintain the newly created sulcus.

Conchal Irregularities

Conchal irregularities may result from injudicious conchal resection, especially from an anterior approach. If a posterior approach is taken, anterior skin excess after isolated conchal cartilage excision may cause unsightly rippling. This usually, but not always, settles with adequate passage of time. Sharp edges may occur within the lateral concha at its junction with the antihelix. Overaggressive resection may also result in an excessively acute angle formed in this location with too severe a medialization of the scaphal element. For these reasons, we prefer a cartilage-sparing approach to conchal setback that combines conchamastoid sutures with posterior mastoid soft tissue resection to allow for retrodisplacement. Tangential shave of the posterior cartilaginous surface eminences may be added without substantial risk of complication if additional setback is needed.

Tragal Prominence

This scenario occurs when a significant conchal setback is attempted without corresponding excision of sufficient postauricular soft tissue to accommodate the conchal retrodisplacement. Thus, persistent postauricular soft tissue exerts anterior and outward counter-pressure on the concha that is, in turn, transmitted to the tragus, increasing its prominence. This condition may co-exist with distortion of the external auditory meatus owing to improper anterior location of conchamastoid sutures. In this scenario, anterior rotation of the concha may lead to impingement of the canal entrance that may adversely affect hearing and the ability to clean the ear canal. This condition is best treated by resection

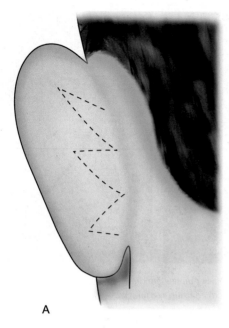

A

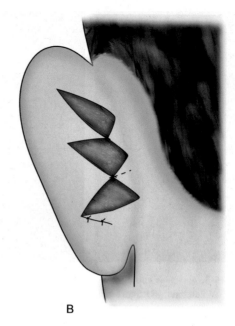

B

Figure 16-6. Treatment of retroauricular sulcus obliteration. (A) Use of a zigzag skin incision within the sulcus. (B) Suturing of the ensuing flaps point-to-point to widen the postauricular sulcus; intervening exposed areas are treated with full thickness skin grafts to prevent excessive contraction.

of the postauricular soft tissues or of the involved medial conchal cartilage via a posterior approach to allow settling of the concha and tragus.

Antitragal or Lobular Prominence

This condition may occur from primary insufficient treatment of a prominent lobule or from loss of correction at the inferior pole involving the cauda helicis. Loss of correction in this area results primarily from injudicious reliance on skin-closing tension to medialize the lobule. Similarly, resection of the cauda helicis may destabilize the lobule and predispose to reprotrusion. A combination of cartilage-shaping techniques and suture techniques may be used to draw the lobule precisely into the desired location. Lobule-mastoid sutures and cauda-conchal sutures may both be utilized effectively for this purpose.

References

1. Richards SD, Jebreel A, Capper R. Otoplasty: a review of the surgical techniques. *Clin Otolaryngol* 30:2–8, 2005.
2. Goode RL, Proffitt SD. Complications of Otoplasty. *Arch Otolaryngol* 1970;91:352–55.
3. Zavod MB, Chen T, Adamson PA. Complications of Otoplasty, Ch. 59. In: Eisele D, Smith R, eds. Com-

plications in Head and Neck Surgery, 2nd edition. Mosby, *In Publication*.
4. Messner AH, Crysdale WS. Otoplasty: clinical protocol and long-term results. *Arch Otolaryngol Head Neck Surg* 122:773–7, 1996.
5. Burstein FD. Cartilage-sparing complete otoplasty technique: a 10-year experience in 100 patients. *J Craniofacial Surg* 14(4):521–5.
6. Calder JC, Naasan A. Morbidity of otoplasty: a retrospective review of 562 consecutive cases. *Br J Plast Surg* 47:170, 1994.
7. Stal S, Spira M. Long-term results in otoplasty. *Facial Plast Surg* 2:153–65, 1985.
8. Adamson PA, McGraw BL, Tropper GJ. Otoplasty: critical review of clinical results. *Laryngoscope* 101: 883, 1991.
9. Stenström SJ, Heftner J. The Stenström otoplasty. *Clin Plast Surg* 5(3):465, 1978.
10. Furnas DW: Complications of surgery of the external ear. *Clin Plast Surg* 17(2):305–318, 1990.
11. Scharer SA, Farrior EH, Farrior RT. Retrospective analysis of the Farrior technique for otoplasty. *Arch Facial Plast Surg* 9:167–73, 2007.
12. Caouette-Laberge L, Guay N, Bortoluzzi P, Belleville C. Otoplasty: anterior scoring technique and results in 500 cases. *Plast Reconstr Surg* 105(2):504–15, 2000.
13. Minderjahn A, Huttl WR, Hildmann H. Mustardé's otoplasty: evaluation of correlation between clini-

cal and statistical findings. *J Max Fac Surg* 8:241, 1980.

14. Manushakian HS, Wilson PA, De Souza BA, McGrouther DA. The prone position in otoplasty. *Plast Reconstr Surg* 115(3):963–4, 2005.

15. Walter C, Nolst Trenité GJ. Revision otoplasty and special problems. *Facial Plast Surg* 10(3):298–308, 1994.

16. Nolst Trenité GJ. Otoplasty: a modified anterior scoring technique. *Facial Plast Surg* 20(4):277–85, 2004.

Index

Information in figures and tables is indicated by *f* and *t*.